Skeletal Radiography

Skeletal Radiography

Sheila Bull
HDCR, TDCR
Senior Tutor, School of Diagnostic Radiography,
Royal Victoria Infirmary, Newcastle upon Tyne

Butterworth
London   Boston   Durban   Singapore   Sydney
Toronto   Wellington

First published 1985

© Butterworth & Co. (Publishers) Ltd, 1985

British Library Cataloguing in Publication Data

Bull, Sheila
   Skeletal radiography.
   1. Skeleton—Radiography
   I. Title
   616.7′10757   RC930.5

   ISBN 0–407–00278–2

Library of Congress Cataloging in Publication Data

Bull, Sheila.
   Skeletal radiography.

   Bibliography: p.
   Includes index.
   1. Radiography, Medical.   I. Title.
   RC78.B83   1985   616.07′572   84-23168
   ISBN 0–407–00277–4
   ISBN 0–407–00278–2 (pbk.)

Typeset by Scribe Design, Gillingham, Kent
Printed and bound in England by Robert Hartnoll Ltd, Bodmin, Cornwall

Preface

The first radiograph was taken in the late nineteenth century and showed the bones of a hand. Since then X-ray technology has progressed remarkably, with the result that modern radiographs are of a quality unimagined by the early pioneers. In keeping with this development, the duties of the radiographer now encompass a wide range of X-ray examinations. These include dealing with highly complex techniques such as digital angiography, computerized tomography and nuclear magnetic resonance imaging. Despite these advances in technology there still remains a strong demand for high-quality 'plain film' radiographs, and a significant portion of this type of work is devoted to radiography of the skeleton. This book is devoted entirely to explaining the modern approach to this traditional branch of radiography.

In terms of coverage, all the relevant radiographic techniques for the skeleton are presented in what is hoped is a clear and easily used fashion. However, it is rarely sufficient to discuss techniques without referring to another important aspect—the reasons why examinations are undertaken and why they are carried out in a particular way. The radiologist may make the final decision as to the precise nature of the pathology present, but the radiographer's skill is inevitably improved if it is supported by an understanding of the nature and outcome of a particular condition. The number of films taken, choice of positioning and exposure factors may be influenced by this additional knowledge. The aim of the book is therefore both to describe skeletal radiographic techniques and to give an outline of some of the more common or noteworthy associated pathologies.

Finally, on a cautionary note, I ask the reader to recognize that there may be several and differing points of view on many topics and, when in doubt, consult other and more specialized works on radiology and pathology.

Acknowledgements

I am grateful to the following consultant radiologists for help and advice: Dr Keith Hall and Dr M.I. Lavelle of the Department of Radiology at the Newcastle Royal Victoria Infirmary; Dr L.N.S. Murthy of the Newcastle Freeman Hospital; and Dr J.P. Owen of the Newcastle University Department of Radiology. I would also like to thank the University Audio Visual Department for the illustrations and in particular Mr Alan Waller who expertly produced the line diagrams. Finally I am indebted to Mrs Kathleen Tunstall, Secretary of the Newcastle Schools of Radiography, and to Mr Richard Whitlock, Teacher Principal of the Newcastle School of Diagnostic Radiography, without whose assistance the writing of this book would have been impossible.

Contents

Part I

Introduction

1

The tissues of the skeleton

Each bone of the skeleton is a complex, living organ made of specialized connective tissue. Collectively they are rigid members of lever systems concerned with body movements and hence they form part of the locomotor system. In addition some bony structures such as the skull and ribs protect vulnerable organs from damage.

Bones also act as a reservoir for certain minerals and play a vital role in the homeostasis of calcium and other ions in the body fluids.

Bone tissue

A characteristic of connective tissues is that they are made up of cells embedded in a matrix of fibres and amorphous (formless) ground substance. In bone the mature cells each lie in a space or lacuna in a collagen matrix heavily impregnated with inorganic minerals collectively known as apatite. This includes calcium and magnesium in combination with phosphate and carbonate. The relatively high atomic number of calcium and the physical density of bone account for its radiopacity as compared with soft tissues. Bone tissue can be classified according to the size of the spaces within it.

Compact (cortical) bone (*Figures 1.1* and *1.2*)

The external covering of a bone (the cortex) is formed by compact bone. In a long bone this layer tends to be thickest in the mid-shaft area and relatively thin over the expanded ends. The cortex appears in a radiograph as a white line

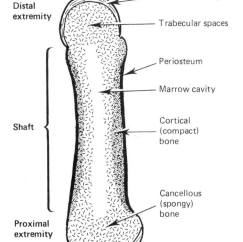

Distal extremity — Hyaline cartilage

— Trabecular spaces

— Periosteum

— Marrow cavity

Cortical (compact) bone

Shaft

Cancellous (spongy) bone

Proximal extremity

Figure 1.1. Diagram of a longitudinal section through a long bone showing its constituent parts. The shaft is formed mainly by a thickened tube of compact bone while the extremities are made of spongy bone with only a thin covering of compact bone

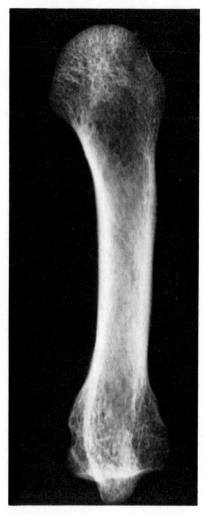

Figure 1.2. Radiograph of a metacarpal. The extremities of the bone take part in the formation of joints and are covered in hyaline cartilage but this covering is not normally visible on the radiograph

Figure 1.3. Schematic diagram of a section through lamellar bone forming the cortex of a tubular (long) bone. The concentric layers of bone surrounding each haversian canal are shown. (Not to scale)

with a sharp and clear outer edge and a less clearly defined inner edge where it merges with the trabeculae of the medulla.

Spongy bone (*Figures 1.1* and *1.2*)

This is also known as trabecular and cancellous bone. The word spongy best describes its appearance—a meshwork of trabeculae (trabeculum means a small beam or bar) surrounded by intercommunicating spaces (cancelli). Spongy bone is found in areas of the skeleton where compressional forces are experienced, e.g. chiefly in the ends of long bones; the bodies of vertebrae; and the calcaneus of the heel. Different types of bone can also be distinguished according to the internal arrangement of fibres and cells.

Lamellar bone

Lamellar means layered, and this type of bone contains haversian systems where concentrically arranged layers of matrix surround a central haversian canal (*Figure 1.3; see* below—The Formation and Growth of Bone). Fine fibre bundles are arranged in these layers in an orderly direction.

Lamellar bone usually replaces cartilage or woven bone in the growing skeleton.

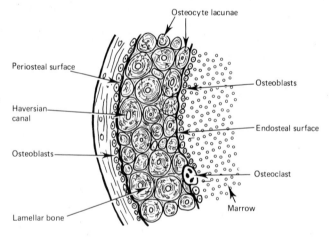

Woven bone

The fibres form an irregular interlacing pattern in a matrix rich in ground substance. The cells are larger than those found in lamellar bone. Woven bone is found wherever bone is rapidly being laid down, e.g. in the embryonic skeleton; subperiosteally in growing bone; in fracture callus (*see* page 15 and 16) and in reactive bone formation in relation to a pathological process. Woven bone is an impermanent structure and is usually replaced by lamellar bone which is mechanically stronger.

Bone cells

Four main types of cell are associated with bone.

(1) *Osteoblasts* which are capable of forming and maintaining bone. They lie on all bone surfaces except those undergoing resorption (*see Figure 1.3*). Osteoblasts are able to respond to stimuli such as changes in the level of parathyroid hormone or calcitonin in the circulation.

(2) *Osteoclasts* are responsible for resorption of bone.

(3) *Osteocytes* are derived from osteoblasts during bone formation. Each osteocyte occupies a lacuna in the bone and gives out cytoplasmic processes which reach out to adjacent areas of bone and also communicate with similar processes derived from osteoblasts (*Figure1.4*). The role of the osteocyte is not entirely understood but they may be responsible for rapid exchanges of calcium between bone and extracellular fluid.

(4) *Fibroblasts* lie on the surface of bone outside the layer of osteoblasts.

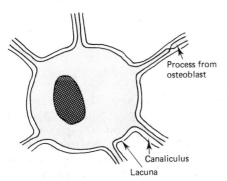

Figure 1.4. Osteocyte cell occupying a lacuna. The cytoplasmic processes communicate via channels known as canaliculi

Bone marrow

The thick cylider of compact bone forming the shaft of a long bone encloses the central marrow cavity which communicates with the cancelli of the spongy bone (*Figure 1.1*). All the spaces are lined with a tissue—the *endosteum*—and are filled with bone marrow which is either fatty or blood forming (haemopoietic). The character of the bone marrow varies with the age of the individual and its location in the skeleton.

Periosteum

This is a tough fibrous membrane that covers the outer surface of the bone except for the articular surface and serves as an attachment for tendons and ligaments (*Figure1.1*).

Between the periosteum and underlying bone lie the osteoblasts (*Figure1.3*) which can become active in bone formation and resorption, and providing that the periosteum remains intact bone formation cannot spread outside it. (Normally the periosteum is not visible on the radiograph.) In certain abnormal conditions the periosteum may become elevated due to haemorrhage as in an injury, or in bone tumours by itself producing new bone (*see Figure 3.12*).

The formation and growth of bone

Most bones, notably long bones, are preformed in hyaline cartilage which is replaced by bone in a process known as ossification. In the fetus the cartilage model is roughly the shape of the future bone (*Figure 1.5a*). A primary ossification zone establishes itself across the width of the shaft and starts extending in both directions towards either end. By birth most of what is later to become the shaft of the bone is ossified but the ends are still cartilaginous (*Figure 1.5b*).

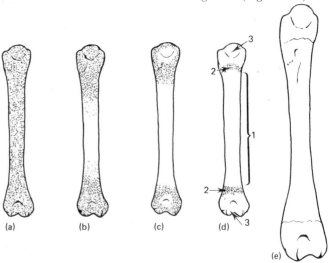

Figure 1.5. Stages of development of a long bone (for key see text)

During the first few years of life secondary ossification centres appear in the cartilaginous ends of the bone (*Figure 1.5c*). Eventually the whole of these extremities are converted to bone except for the articular surfaces which remain covered by cartilage. A thin zone of cartilage also persists between the ends of the bone and its shaft (*Figure 1.5d*). It is at these growth or epiphyseal plates and adjacent part of the shaft that a long bone will continue to increase in length.

The terms used for the parts of the growing bone are (*Figure 1.5*):

1. Diaphysis.
2. Epiphyseal plate.
3. Epiphysis.

A long bone grows in length by the interstitial growth of the epiphyseal plate cartilage in which the cells (chondrocytes) are arranged in columns lying parallel to the longitudinal axis of the bone. These columns or palisades are produced by repeated cell division. Each row of cells is surrounded by cartilage matrix with thin partitions lying between the cells. As the cells approach the diaphyseal side of the plate they enlarge and the matrix in which they are enclosed becomes calcified. Cells next to the marrow cavity die and the thin transverse partitions of matrix disappear leaving tunnels which are invaded by capillaries and osteoblasts. The osteoblasts put down several layers of bone (lamellae) on the inner walls of the tunnels and this process is repeated until only a narrow channel (haversian canal) containing a neurovascular bundle remains. Bone-forming cells are now entrapped in their lacunae in the newly formed layers of bone. The cells are now termed osteocytes.

Each concentric arrangement of layers of bone matrix and cells is called an haversian system. The narrow canaliculi containing the cell cytoplasmic processes pass radially and circumferentially in the haversian systems conveying nutrient to the enclosed osteocytes (*see Figures 1.3 and 1.4*).

During the growing period the interstitial growth of the epiphyseal cartilage keeps pace with its replacement by bone so the epiphyseal plate is always present as a thin, radiolucent zone. The actively growing part of the diaphysis adjacent to the epiphyseal cartilage is known as the *metaphysis*. Fusion of the plate with its neighbouring bony elements halts any further increase in bone length. When this occurs the bone is said to have reached maturity (*Figure 1.5e*). Growth in width in a long bone and growth in all other bones is achieved by deposition of new bone on the periosteal and endosteal surfaces of the existing bone— *appositional* growth.

Conversion of cartilage to bone is known as *endochondral ossification*. A few bony elements notably the clavicle and the bones of the skull vault are formed by ossification of connective tissue membranes (mesenchyme). This is known as *intramembranous ossification*.

Measuring the stage of bone maturity

The radiographic appearance (or non-appearance) of the ossification centres in a limb can be used as an indicator of the stage of skeletal maturity.

In 1937 an *Atlas of Skeletal Maturation of the Hand* was published, later to be revised by Greulich and Pyle[1]. This work recognized the importance of serial changes of maturing ossification centres which were considered to be maturity determinators. Posterior-anterior hand and wrist radiographs can be taken and compared with the atlas. A skeletal age differing from chronological age by more than one year is generally regarded as lying outside normal limits[2].

In 1967 Tanner, Whitehouse and Healy produced a new method for assessing skeletal maturity that was believed to be more flexible and derived from a more solid mathematical base. In this system each bone of the hand and wrist was classified separately into one of eight or nine stages, to which scores were assigned. These scores were summed to give skeletal maturity. This system has subsequently been revised and the new approach provides separate maturities for the carpal bones and the long bones[3].

The determination of skeletal maturity may be used in the diagnosis and treatment of endocrine disorders in children, in the prediction of adult height and in general surveys for public health purposes.

Bone remodelling and turnover

Bone tissue is not static; it is constantly being produced and destroyed. In the process of *remodelling*, bone tissue is deposited on some surfaces whilst it is removed from others. This turnover rate is much faster in growing bone whose interior structure is changing continually to adjust to increasing size and shape. The effects of remodelling are

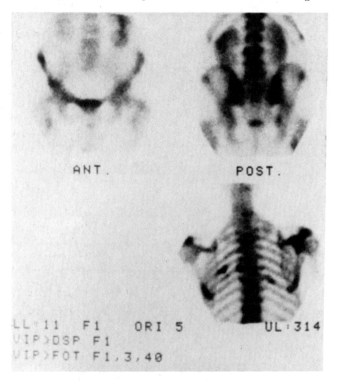

Figure 1.6. The image produced in radioisotope scintigraphy of bone. The patient has myelomatosis (*see* Chapter 3). Note areas of increased activity in the ribs where foci of bone destruction are present

more startling, for example, in a child with a fracture that has healed with deformity—the deformity is seen to diminish gradually and the bone returns to its 'normal' shape (*see* Chapter 2). Even in the adult, bone is continually being remodelled. Accretion and resorption occur simultaneously and each process uses about 500 mg of calcium daily.

Studies with radioactive isotopes have shown that there is a pool of readily exchangeable calcium within the bone[4]. The anatomical site of this pool is not clear but it has been estimated that bone crystal surfaces exposed to extracellular fluid on the walls of the lacunae, canaliculi and haversian canals amount to 1500–5000 m^2 on average. The continual exchange of the mineral between bone and the extracellular fluid is illustrated by the use of radioisotope scintigraphy (*Figure 1.6*). This technique may be used to indicate areas of the skeleton with increased turnover such as the sites of bony secondaries in malignant disease; increased turnover is also seen where there is healing of fractures or at the growing ends of normal bone in children.

Joints of the skeleton

Joints are functional connections between different bones of the skeleton, and they can be classified according to their structure and degree of movement. The major moving joints of the body are those that have a joint cavity. These are termed *diarthroses*.

The ends of the bones forming the articulation are almost invariably covered by hyaline cartilage which is some 2–4 mm thick (in the young). The cartilage's normal radiolucency provides the effective 'joint space' seen on the radiograph. When damaged, articular cartilage has little power of regeneration.

The joint surfaces are lubricated and the cartilage nourished by synovial fluid. Normal human joints contain less than 1 ml of this fluid and a large intra-articular accumulation is termed an *effusion*.

Structural support for the bone ends is provided for by the strong surrounding *fibrous capsule* reinforced by localized thickenings—*ligaments*—and adjacent structures such as tendons or muscles.

Joints where the bone margins are united by a layer of fibrous tissue are called fibrous joints. Because they are 'immovable' they are also termed *synarthroses*. Examples of fibrous joints include the sutures of the skull.

A third type of joint is known as an *amphiarthrosis* or 'slightly' moving joint and in this case the bone ends are united by cartilage. Examples of these cartilaginous joints include those that lie between the pubic bones and between the vertebral bodies. In both of these locations the bone joint surfaces are covered in hyaline cartilage and separated by a disc of fibrocartilage.

Ligaments and tendons

Ligaments are designed to prevent the occurrence of excessive or abnormal movements at joints and tendons are integral parts of the extremities of skeletal muscles. Both are made of dense, fibrous connective tissue and are attached to bone at their origins and insertions by an interweaving of the collagen fibres with those of the periosteum. Sharpey's fibres extend from the ligaments and tendons through the periosteum into the substance of the underlying cortical bone. In certain injuries of a tendon or ligament a portion of cortical bone may be pulled away or *avulsed* from the main body of bone due to the firm anchorage provided by Sharpey's fibres (*see* Chapter 2—avulsion fracture).

References

1. GRUELICH, W.W. and PYLE, S.I. (1959). *Radiographic Atlas of Skeletal Development of the Hand and Wrist.* California; Stanford University Press.
2. EDEIKEN, J. and HODES, P.J. (1973). *Roentgen Diagnosis of Diseases of Bone,* p. 18. Baltimore; Williams and Williams.
3. TANNER, J.M., WHITEHOUSE, R.H., MARSHALL, W.A., HEALEY, M.J.B. and GOLDSTEIN, H. (1975). *Assessment of Skeletal Maturity and Prediction of Adult Height.* London; Academic Press.
4. BELL, G.H., EMSLIE-SMITH, D. and PATERSON, C.R. (1980). *Textbook of Physiology.* Edinburgh; Churchill Livingstone.

2 Fractures and dislocations

The most common request for radiography of the skeleton is made because of the need to exclude or confirm the presence of a bony injury.

Fractures of bone

A fracture is a break in the continuity of bone and the bone pieces are referred to as fragments. Any break, even of one cortex constitutes a fracture. Fractures are said to be either *simple* or *compound*.

Simple fractures

In a simple fracture there is no direct communication between the fracture and the external environment.

Compound fractures

In a compound fracture there is a direct communication between the fracture and the skin surface, e.g. a fracture of the tibia with a laceration of the overlying skin. Compound fractures are likely to become infected while simple fractures are not.

Several other terms are used to describe fractures:

(1) Comminuted—more than two fragments are present (*Figure 2.1*).
(2) Greenstick—an incomplete break occurring in children whose bones are 'soft'. On the X-ray film the bone may be seen to be buckled (*Figure 2.2*).

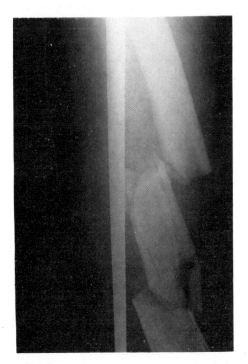

Figure 2.1. A comminuted fracture of the lower femur

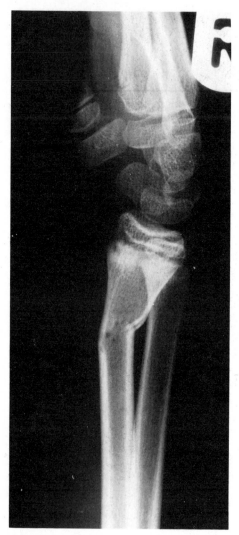

Figure 2.2. A greenstick fracture of the lower end of the radius. The ulnar styloid process is also fractured

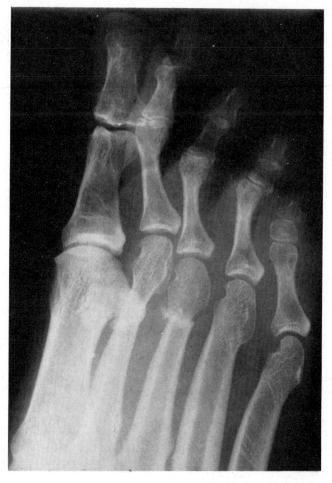

Figure 2.3. A stress fracture (march fracture—*see* Chapter 7) through the neck of the third metatarsal

(3) Avulsion—usually caused by traction of the tendon tearing off a bone fragment at the point of its insertion.

(4) Stress—similar to fatigue fractures in metal; this type of fracture results from repeated application of a minor force (*Figure 2.3*).

(5) Complicated—all fractures involve some soft tissue damage. In complicated fractures there is also damage to some important structure such as a nerve, vessel or viscus (*Figure 2.4*).

(6) Pathological—a fracture occurring through abnormal bone, e.g. at the site of a secondary deposit from a carcinoma (*Figure 2.5*).

(7) Crush—where cancellous bone has collapsed owing to compressive forces, e.g. in a *wedge fracture* of a vertebral body (*see* Chapter 8).

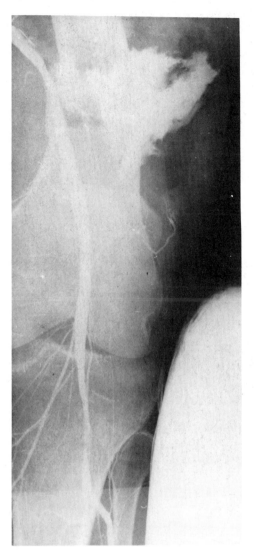

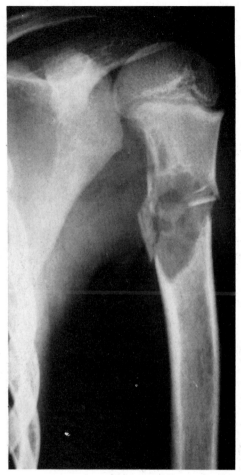

Figure 2.5. A pathological fracture through an osteolytic (bone-destroying) lesion in the upper humerus

Figure 2.4. A comminuted fracture of the lower femur which is also complicated by injury to the popliteal artery. Contrast agent is leaking from the damaged blood vessel

The orientation and state of the fracture line are described by further terms such as *transverse, oblique* or *spiral*. Where the fragments are driven into each other the fracture is said to be *impacted*.

The type and direction of the applied force may have some influence on the way in which the bone breaks. If the injuring force is applied directly to the bone then the fracture is more likely to be of the comminuted type and possibly compound. The transmission of violence, e.g. by a twisting of the limb, may cause a spiral or oblique fracture.

Fractures in children

The epiphysis can be separated from the diaphysis forcefully. This is known as *fracture separation* or *displacement* of the epiphysis. It occurs in children when an equivalent force would produce a fracture in adults.

Signs and symptoms of a fracture

The radiographer should be aware of the signs and symptoms of a fracture. These may affect the degree of co-operation the patient can achieve and hence alter the approach to the radiographic technique.

The patient will be in pain and may lose function of the limb. The fracture site itself is painful. The limb may look deformed, owing to displacement, angulation or overlapping of the fragments. There could also be abnormal mobility at the fracture or even crepitus of the fragment ends.

Treatment

The orthopaedic surgeon will make clinical judgements in the management of a fracture. The function of radiography is to aid assessment before, during and after treatment. Radiographs can easily show bony alignment and may reveal information concerning the degree and success of the fracture healing.

Reduction

First of all the fragments are replaced in their proper alignment. The term 'reduction' refers to the normalizing of any angulation or displacement present. Not all fractures need 'reducing'. Reduction takes place under some form of anaesthetic. If the surgeon has to operate and expose the bone fragments before they are re-aligned then this is known as *open reduction*.

Immobilization or fixation

The bone ends must now be held firmly in apposition until the fragments stick together or *unite*.

External fixation

This includes fixation by
(1) Splints, which are usually made of metal or plastic and held on by bandages.
(2) Plaster of Paris casts.
(3) Traction. This works by applying a pulling force along the line of the limb to hold the two fragments in position. Where the force is slowly applied over a period of time, traction can be used to *reduce* a fracture or dislocation.

Internal fixation

This is the use of special metal 'implants' to hold the bone fragments together. The advantage of this method is that it

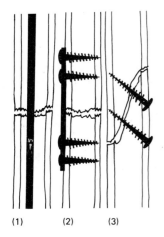

(1) (2) (3)

Figure 2.6. Types of metal implant used in internal fixation of fractures

allows earlier mobilization of the patient. Many types of internal fixation devices are available, all of which are scientifically designed and utilize advanced engineering principles.

Materials in use are high grade stainless steel and various alloys of chrome, cobalt, molybdenum, tungsten and nickel. There are three main types of implant (*Figure 2.6*)

(1) Intramedullary rods and wires—these are used for long bones.

(2) Plates held on with screws.

(3) Screws to hold fragments together.

The pin and plate used for trochanteric fractures of the femur is a combination of intramedullary pin for the femoral neck and a plate for the shaft.

The healing process of bone (*Figure 2.7*)

(1) Immediately after the injury the fracture bleeds and a clot is formed. This haematoma acts as a bridge along which cells grow.

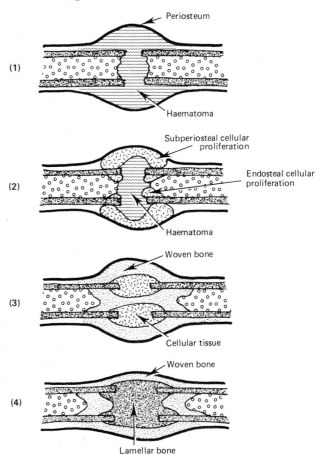

Figure 2.7. Stages in the process of fracture healing

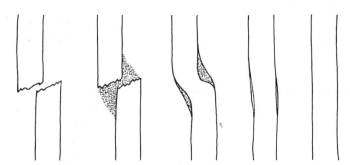

Figure 2.8. Remodelling of a bone after a fracture

(2) Osteoblasts from the periosteum and endosteum form a collar of cellular tissue which soon grows to link the ends of both fragments. The haematoma gradually disappears.

(3) The active osteoblasts lay down intercellular matrix (osteoid) which becomes impregnated with calcium salts to form primitive woven bone. Calcified woven bone (callus) is visible on the radiograph.

(4) The woven bone is eventually replaced by mature lamellar or haversian bone. During this last stage of consolidation, *remodelling* of the bone takes place (*Figures 2.8 and 2.9*). This means that the callus collar is removed and the bone is effectively reshaped by the action of osteoblasts and osteoclasts. In children remodelling after a fracture is

Figure 2.9. A fracture of the tibia and fibula (*a*) at the time of injury (*b*) during the later stages of healing

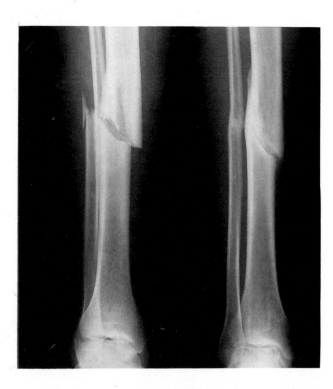

often so perfect that the site becomes indistinguishable on the X-ray films.

Union of the fragments

The fracture is said to be united when the bone moves as a single unit and is not tender when gently stressed. This is a clinical sign and is not always linked with the appearances on the radiograph. *Radiological union* is when the cortices of the (two) fragments are seen to be joined on the radiograph.

The time scale for healing varies.

Young children—4–6 weeks to reach consolidation.
Adults   —3–5 months.

Union may be delayed for a variety of reasons such as restricted blood supply to the fracture site, local infection or inadequate fixation or immobilization. If the bone fails to unite then healing may be stimulated by *bone grafting*. On the other hand the fragments may unite in the 'wrong' position. This is called *mal-union*.

Rehabilitation

Once the fracture has united treatment may continue so that the patient regains full use of the limb. The fracture may have to be protected for a while especially if it is a weight bearing limb.

Appliances to perform this job include crutches, splints and calipers. Graduated exercises (physiotherapy) are then undertaken to build up muscles that have become wasted owing to disuse.

Joint injuries

Sprains

This is a tearing of the joint capsule or its supporting ligaments. The only radiological evidence of this may be soft tissue swelling over the affected area.

Subluxations

A subluxation is a partial displacement of the articular surface of a joint, with the bones still remaining in contact with each other. These occur most commonly in the 'plane' variety of synovial joints such as the acromioclavicular.

Dislocations (luxations)

This is a complete separation of the articular surfaces of a joint as the result of trauma. The joint capsule is often extensively torn. Pathological dislocation may occur where there is some abnormal muscle pull or where the joint has been destroyed by some pathological process.

Fracture dislocations

A fracture dislocation is a combination injury where the bone is fractured at the same time as it is dislocated. These are most frequently seen in severe injuries of the ankle and the elbow joints.

3 Pathological conditions of bones and joints

Disease may be defined as an abnormal variation in the structure and function of any part of the body, and pathology can be described as the scientific study of disease.

Many factors are known to influence and modify bone production and development. For example, deprivation or excess of raw materials, vitamins and hormonal imbalances can each result in abnormalities. However, there are many diseases of bones and joints for which the causes are not clearly understood.

The radiographer will be required to carry out X-ray examinations of the skeleton to exclude or assess the extent of an abnormality. A radiograph of a normal bone will demonstrate its normal anatomy and normal mineralization. If the rate of bone formation or destruction becomes significantly altered by some pathological process then this abnormality may become detectable on a radiograph. For example, there may be visible changes in the thickness or physical density of the bone's cortex or alterations in the trabecular pattern (*Figures 3.1* and *3.2*). It should not be forgotten, however, that many soft-tissue abnormalities may also be shown on radiographs that have been taken principally to exclude skeletal pathology. The radiographer may be required to carry out X-ray examinations of the skeleton as part of several investigations in the clinical management of patients.

The remainder of this chapter contains brief descriptions of some of the more common or well-known pathological conditions of bone and joints. These conditions are mostly of a generalized nature, i.e. they can affect several bones or joints or even the whole of the skeleton at any one time. Some of the diseases are not necessarily of a generalized nature but could still occur at any location of the skeleton, e.g. neoplastic conditions, osteoarthritis. Further comments on these conditions when they affect certain specific areas of the skeleton may be found in Part II.

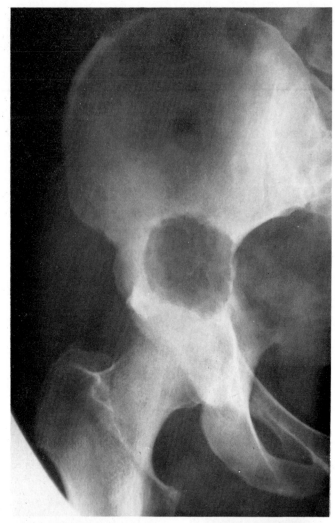

Figure 3.1. A well-demarcated osteolytic (bone-destroying) lesion in the innominate bone

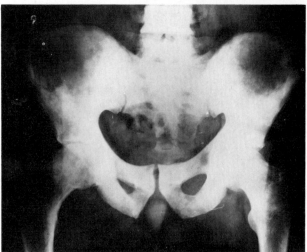

Figure 3.2. Osteopetrosis affecting the pelvis. The radiographic appearance implies that the physical density of the bone is much greater than normal

Diseases of bone due to vitamin deficiency

Vitamin D deficiency

Bone is built in two stages:

(1) Osteoblasts lay down intercellular substance or matrix (osteoid) which is not radiopaque.
(2) Salts of calcium and phosphorus are later deposited to form true bone.

Deficiency in vitamin D results in an increase in the proportion of uncalcified osteoid present. In adults this produces a condition known as *osteomalacia* and in the growing skeleton of infants and children results in *rickets*.

Causes of vitamin D deficiency include:

(1) Low dietary intake of vitamin D combined with little exposure to sunlight.
(2) Malabsorption syndromes.
(3) Renal failure.

Osteomalacia

The outcome of lack of mineralization of the bone is weakness with a tendency to deformation and pathological fractures—*milkman's fractures*—which are usually symmetrical. Radiographs may show linear areas of increased radiolucency—*Looser's zones* (*Figure 3.3*)—and are particularly common in the pubic rami, inner scapular borders, neck of humerus and medial aspects of the femoral shafts. Some patients may have only a generalized decrease in bone density (which may not even be detected by radiographs), especially noticeable in the peripheral skeleton when compared with the spine.

For patients with long-standing renal disease such as those on renal dialysis, *renal osteodystrophy* is a term that embraces a resultant complex of changes in the skeleton. These can include osteomalacia (rickets in a child), secondary hyperparathyroidism (*see* below) and osteosclerosis. Soft-tissue and vascular calcifications can occur.

Patients undergoing renal dialysis are usually monitored for these bony changes with periodic radiographic surveys.

Rickets (Figure 3.4)

Rickets is characterized by failure in the mineralization of osteoid bone and a failure of mineralization of the cartilage of the epiphyseal growth plate. Radiographs of long bone show expansion and cupping of the metaphyseal regions so that the diaphysis appears to expand into the shape of a trumpet-mouth at the metaphysis. The bone shafts lose rigidity because of the failure in mineralization and deformities and fractures can occur.

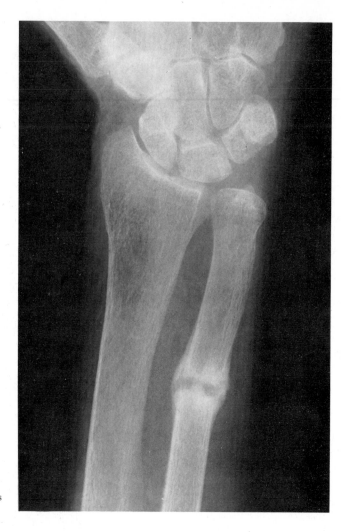

Figure 3.3. Characteristic appearance of a Looser's zone in the right ulna

Vitamin C deficiency

Vitamin C is important in the synthesis of collagen which is formed in the metaphyses of bone and in the walls of blood vessels. Deficiency of vitamin C causes scurvy. In very young children large haematomas may form under the periosteum in response to relatively minor trauma. The osteoblasts on the under-surface proceed to form new bone and considerable time is required for remodelling to occur. Similar haematomas with ossification may be seen on radiographs of the bones of 'battered babies' (*see* Chapter 12). In adults, particularly elderly males who live alone, scurvy is dominated by changes of capillary fragility in the skin and mucous membrane; there are rarely any skeletal radiological signs.

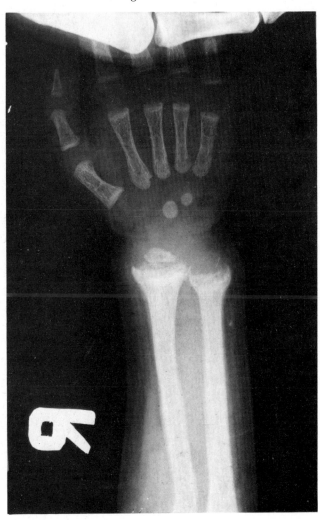

Figure 3.4. Characteristic appearance of rickets in the forearm bones of a child

Changes in bone due to endocrine disorders

Growth hormone oversecretion

Two conditions are the result of prolonged and excessive secretion of growth hormone which is usually caused by the presence of a tumour in the pituitary gland—*acidophil adenoma*.

The lateral skull radiograph may show an increase in the size of the pituitary fossa due to the tumour.

Acromegaly (Figure 3.5)

This means 'enlargement of the extremities' although other parts of the skeleton are affected. This condition occurs in

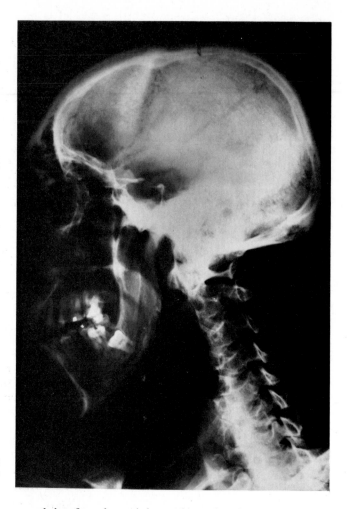

Figure 3.5. Acromegaly. Lateral radiograph of the skull and face, showing a notable increase in the size of the jaw. The pituitary fossa is also enlarged

an adult after the epiphyses have fused so although the bones cannot elongate they can grow thicker by periosteal ossification. There is an increase in the roughening of the surfaces of the bones and of the sites of insertion of tendons, and irregular bone growth distorts the joint surfaces so that osteoarthritis commonly results. Changes in the skull also occur—the orbital ridges enlarge and prognathism (protrusion of the mandible) may occur.

Gigantism

This is a much rarer condition and occurs where there is oversecretion of growth hormone before the epiphyses have fused. There is an increased growth of the whole skeleton and growth may continue for longer than normal because of delay in closure of the epiphyseal plates.

Parathyroid hyperfunction

Plasma calcium ion concentrations are maintained within narrow limits (mineral homeostasis) because this is necessary for normal function of muscles and nerves and for the activities of several enzymes. Normally, calcium is constantly entering the blood plasma from bone and gut; and leaving it for bone, gut or to be excreted in the urine. The principal action of parathyroid hormone (PTH) is to increase the resorption of calcium in the renal tubules. Higher concentrations of PTH in the plasma stimulate resorption of bone by osteoclasts and indirectly increase calcium absorption from the gut. Thus PTH has an important role in the regulation of plasma calcium levels. An excess of PTH in the blood can produce symptoms associated with the action of the hormone in a condition known as *hyperparathyroidism.*

Hyperparathyroidism can be classified as primary, secondary and tertiary. Whatever the cause of the hyperparathyroidism, one skeletal feature is common—the appearance of the surface resorption of bone by osteoclasts. These changes are called sub-periosteal erosions and are best shown by radiography of the fingers.

Primary hyperparathyroidism

In primary hyperparathyroidism there is excessive PTH secretion, which is usually due to a tumour involving one or more of the parathyroid glands. The patient may develop kidney stones, and calcium salts may be deposited in the walls of blood vessels. Symptoms relating to bone changes are not frequent—they are recognizable in only 10–20% of patients. Over a period of time these changes can range from a generalized diminution in bone density to cyst formation.

Secondary hyperparathyroidism

This occurs when the glands are exposed to increased stimulation to produce PTH as a compensatory reaction to *hypocalcaemia* which can occur in chronic renal failure and in untreated malabsorption syndromes.

Tertiary hyperparathyroidism

In secondary hyperparathyroidism an autonomous, usually benign parathyroid tumour may develop. If this happens then the hyperparathyroidism is no longer compensatory and is termed tertiary hyperparathyroidism.

Hypothyroidism

Undersecretion of thyroid hormone may occur at any age. In adults this causes *myxoedema.* If the deficiency is present at birth then the result will be a condition called *cretinism.*

The child's skeletal and mental development will be retarded. Often the earliest clue is the late appearance of secondary ossification centres in the epiphyses, e.g. of the hands, lower femur or upper tibia; when they do appear growth is retarded and the centres are often fragmented.

Miscellaneous conditions of bone

Osteoporosis (*Figure 3.6*)

This is a condition where there is a decrease in the total amount of bone present, the remaining bone containing normal amounts of minerals. The cause could be either an acceleration in bone tissue resorption or a decrease in bone formation. Radiographic detection depends upon the amount of bone that has been lost; as bone mass diminishes radiopacity will decrease. Variations between individuals

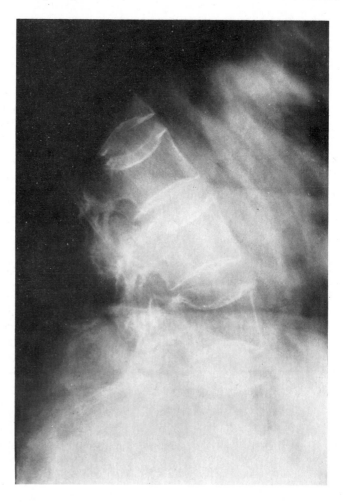

Figure 3.6. 'Cod-fish' vertebrae in osteoporosis. ...ck of radiographic contrast is caused by the ...ninution of the total amount of bone tissue present

and variations in radiographic technique can make evaluation of bone density difficult and in general radiology is not very sensitive in this disease. Often considerable loss of bone must occur before it is seen on the radiograph. In patients with advanced osteoporosis a fairly large decrease in exposure may be required to produce an image of relatively acceptable photographic density and contrast.

The radiological signs that have been attributed to osteoporosis are thinning of the cortical bone with loss of bony trabeculae. The resultant effects of reduction in bone strength may be seen in the spine. The nucleus pulposus inside the vertebral body is normally under pressure. As the bone of the vertebral body loses strength the disc tends to become more spherical. The bone collapses under the expansive force of the nucleus which allows the discs to become biconvex and produces biconcave vertebral bodies—*cod-fish vertebrae* (*Figure 3.6*). Weakening of bones in osteoporosis can make them more vulnerable to fractures.

The causes of osteoporosis include the following:

(1) Old age—*senile osteoporosis* tends to affect women more than men.
(2) Prolonged immobilization. Bone responds to increased use by making itself better able to withstand the greater mechanical stresses. Osteoblasts build more numerous and wider trabeculae. Conversely, disuse can lead to fewer, thin and frail trabeculae as in *disuse* osteoporosis.
(3) *Steroid* therapy. Steroids affect the trabecular bone and induce osteoporosis. Osteoporosis can also be found in Cushing's disease.
(4) Excess thyroid hormone—*thyrotoxicosis*. There is an increase of both resorption and bone formation but resorption exceeds formation.

Paget's disease of bone (osteitis deformans)

This disease of unknown cause occurs in the middle aged and elderly, usually after the age of 40, and is more common in men than in women and more common in certain races.

The areas of the skeleton most frequently affected are the lumbar vertebrae, skull and pelvis, although limb bones may also be involved. The affected bone becomes larger than normal and on the radiograph the texture of the bone becomes more coarse. Deformities such as bowing of the long bones or kyphosis of the dorsal spine can occur.

If the skull is affected the bones of the vault will increase in thickness, causing an increase in the size of the patient's head (*see Figure 10.6*). Involvement of the base of the skull may cause nerve entrapment, and deafness is not uncommon. Other complications of Paget's disease are pathological fractures, malignant changes in the bone and heart failure because of the strain of an increased blood flow through the affected area (this may be up to 20 times the normal).

Fibrous dysplasia of bone

Fibrous dysplasia is characterized by fibrous replacement of portions of the medullary cavity of bone or bones. The cause of the disease is unknown and it begins in young individuals, often in infancy, but because it is asymptomatic it often remains unrecognized until adulthood.

Avascular necrosis of bone

Owing to the vascular anatomy at particular sites, fractures may be complicated by severance of the blood supply to one of the bony fragments. This results in degeneration of the fragment. In other cases of avascular necrosis, trauma is not an obvious cause. An example of this is necrosis of bone encountered in divers and compressed-air workers (*see* Chapter 12).

In children and adolescents osteonecrosis occurs at several epiphyseal sites for no known cause (although there may be repeated minor trauma in some cases). A cycle of changes can be seen and followed in serial radiographs. The avascular bone becomes relatively more dense than its neighbours. The dead bone then begins to crumble and collapse. Later the area becomes revascularized and its abnormal density disappears. The dead bone is removed and new bone laid down in its place, but owing to softening the shape is now distorted. The general name for this condition is *juvenile osteochondritis* or simply *osteochondritis* and various eponymous terms are applied according to the site affected:

(1) Femoral head—Perthe's disease.
(2) Ring epiphysis of vertebral bodies—Scheuermann's disease.
(3) Tibial tubercle—Osgood–Schlatter's disease.
(4) Head of 2nd or 3rd metatarsal—Freiberg's disease.
(5) Calcaneus—Sever's disease.
(6) Navicular—Köhler's disease.
(7) Lunate—Kienböck's disease.

Osteochondritis dissecans

Essentially this consists of the necrosis of an area of bone adjacent to a joint surface with accompanying death of the deeper layers of its covering cartilage. Hence this segment of the articular surface may become separated and form a *loose body* inside the joint cavity.

Areas most commonly affected are the knee, elbow and ankle. As the disease usually occurs towards the end of the growing period, osteochondritis dissecans is seen predominantly in adolescents and young adults.

Generalized developmental abnormalities

Osteopetrosis (*see Figure 3.2*)

This is a rare condition characterized by brittle bones which on the X-ray film are shown to be excessively dense (*see Figure 3.2*). In addition to increased brittleness, the condition causes depression of the marrow function and compression of cranial nerves within the base of the skull.

Osteogenesis imperfecta (*Figure 3.7*)

Osteogenesis imperfecta is a rare congenital disorder where there is abnormal fragility or brittleness of bones. The cortical bone is thin and defective and the patient may suffer from multiple fractures.

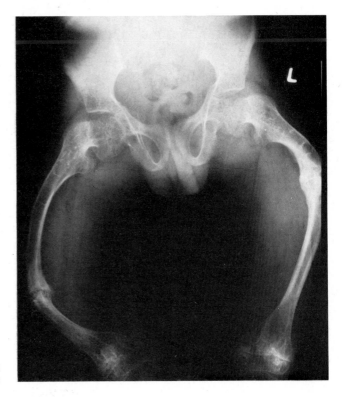

Figure 3.7. Osteogenesis imperfecta. The femora are deformed and contain healing pathological fractures

Achondroplasia (*Figure 3.8*)

Achondroplasia is one of the causes of severe dwarfing; a hereditary defect of 'pre-bone' cartilage in which the normal formation of cartilage cells during bone growth does not occur—hence the long bones cannot grow to their correct length. The periosteal bone formation is normal so

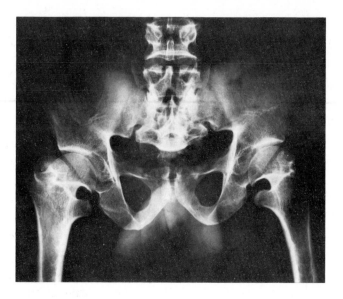

Figure 3.8. The pelvis of an adult affected by achondroplasia

the resulting bone is short but thick and strong. The child will have a normal trunk and short limbs. Because the vault of the skull is formed from membranous bone it increases in size, whereas the base of the skull and the face are formed from cartilage bone and do not develop to the same extent—the base of the skull tends to be flat.

Multiple exostosis

This is a condition where there is a failure of the normal progress of remodelling of the metaphyseal region of long bones and a presence of exostoses arising from the metaphysis. The main bones affected are the femur, tibia, ulna, radius and humerus.

Infections of bone

Bone is liable to infections like any other tissue. Organisms may reach the bone either directly through a skin wound in a compound fracture, or indirectly via the bloodstream. Organisms common in bone infections are *Staphylococcus aureus* and salmonellae.

Acute haematogenous osteomyelitis

This is a bacterial infection arising in the metaphyseal region of the bone, most often a disease of children and usually affecting the bone before epiphyseal lines have closed.

The infection reaches the metaphyseal region via the bloodstream from a septic focus elsewhere in the body, e.g. a boil. Once established the infection spreads in various directions into the surrounding bone and neighbouring parts. A sub-periosteal abscess is formed and deprives the underlying bone of a blood supply—this segment of bone dies and eventually separates to form a *sequestrum*.

As the disease progresses the elevated periosteum lays down layers of new bone, an *involucrum*. Eventually the abscess bursts through the periosteum and spreads to the surface to form a chronic sinus.

Chronic osteomyelitis

This relapsing type of osteomyelitis can follow an acute attack, which suggests that the original infection has not completely responded to treatment. The causative organisms can lie dormant in certain parts of the affected area and they occasionally become reactivated. Sinus tracks may be investigated by injection of a radiopaque contrast agent in *sinography*.

Brodie's abscess

This is a persistent abscess in the metaphyseal region of a bone and appears to develop without a preceding attack. Treatment comprises opening and emptying the cavity. If the abscess cavity is small it may be pin-pointed before incision by insertion of a guide-wire under X-ray control.

Tuberculosis of bone and joint (*see Figure 3.9*)

The commonest and most important type of chronic infection of bone is that due to tuberculosis. In the UK within the past 20 years the number of cases has diminished. It still remains common in the developing countries and during the past few years there have been occasional cases within the immigrant population in the UK. The causative organism (*Mycobacterium tuberculosis*) reaches the bone via the bloodstream from a primary focus either in the lungs or in the alimentary tract. This initial site of infection may still be active or may be healed by the time the skeletal focus is discovered. Tuberculous bacilli may infect primarily bone or synovial membrane but usually both the joint and neighbouring bones are eventually affected (*Figure 3.9*).

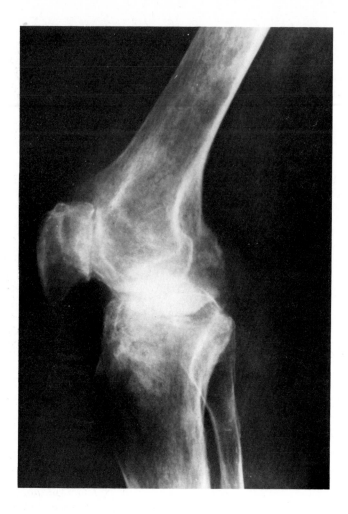

Figure 3.9. Tuberculosis affecting the knee joint

Miscellaneous joint conditions

Osteoarthritis (degenerative arthrosis)

The old term for degeneration of joints is osteoarthritis. In recent years *osteoarthrosis* has found favour mainly because in this condition the joint is not necessarily inflamed, which the word-ending 'itis' would seem to suggest. There are two main types:

(1) *Primary osteoarthritis*—Where there is no known cause for the degeneration; several joints may be affected simultaneously.
(2) *Secondary osteoarthritis*—Where there has been previous destruction of articular cartilage or disruption of the joint surfaces, e.g. following a fracture.

Osteoarthritis is the commonest form of chronic joint disease and is characterized clinically by the progressive

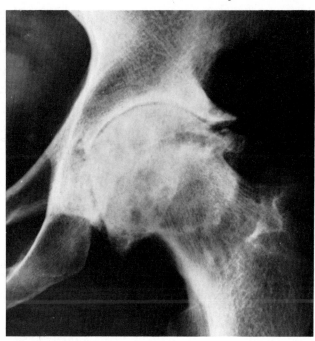

Figure 3.10. Osteoarthritis in the left hip joint

onset of joint pain and stiffness. This causes most problems when it affects the weight-bearing joints—hips, knees and ankles. The patients are usually elderly and the radiographer may have to adapt the technique to suit a patient with limited movement. The typical radiological appearances of osteoarthritis (*Figure 3.10*) are:

(1) The joint space becomes narrowed.
(2) Osteophytes (bony growths) are formed. Where the synovial membrane joins the articular surface the cartilage hypertrophies and spreads a little way into the capsule. Cartilaginous excrescences are in time converted to bone giving rise to osteophytes.
(3) Juxta-articular sclerosis.

Degenerative joint disease can be treated by operation, as follows.

Arthrodesis—The joint is permanently stiffened. This gives complete relief of pain but may throw increased strain on other joints.

Osteotomy—The pain of arthritis can usually be relieved by cutting across the bone distal to the joint and then allowing it to unite in a slightly altered position. The bone is fixed internally until it has united. Osteotomy can be used to correct deformities caused either by degeneration *or* following mal-union of a fracture.

Arthroplasty—Making a new joint. There are several methods, e.g. one or both bony components of the joint are excised and replaced by a metal or plastic prosthesis (substitute). The joints most commonly treated are the knee (e.g. Freeman–Swanson prosthesis) and the hip (Charnley total hip prosthesis and its variants)—*see* Chapter 7.

Rheumatoid disease

This is a general systemic disease which can involve many body organs. However, changes in the joints—*rheumatoid arthritis*—is usually the dominant feature. The disease tends to affect more than one joint and usually starts in the small joints of the hands and feet but can affect the larger joints such as the knee. The joints become inflamed and swollen—this often spontaneously resolves but sometimes the disease can progress leading to disorganization of the joints and development of deformities.

Ankylosing spondylitis (*Figure 3.11*)

This is a progressive stiffening of the spine starting in the lumbar region and moving upwards. Ossification of the

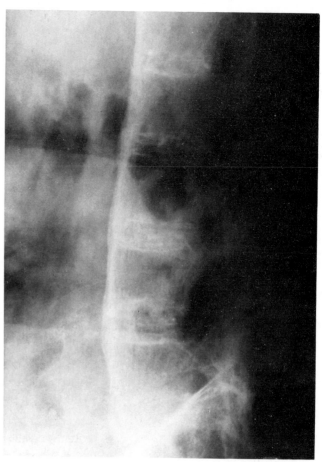

Figure 3.11. Lateral radiograph of the lumbar spine showing ankylosing spondylitis

surrounding soft tissues and lateral bony bridging of the vertebrae give rise to a radiographic appearance after which the disease is sometimes named—*bamboo spine*.

Stiffening of the spine/rib joints restrict the patient's breathing volume because of the limiting of chest expansion. If untreated the patient may end up with a severe rigid flexion deformity of the spine and neck which is very disabling.

The earliest changes in ankylosing spondylitis are seen in the sacroiliac joints; in the rest of the spine changes may not be seen until much later. In severe cases the disease may also involve the shoulders, hips, knees and occasionally the temporomandibular joints. This disease also can affect the eyes in *iritis* and other organs of the body more rarely.

Loose bodies in joints

Smooth movement of a joint may be upset by the presence of a piece of bone or cartilage lying free in the joint space. The fragment has probably separated from one of the joint surfaces but its presence is not suspected until the joint suddenly locks or its range of flexion is reduced. Where there is sudden interference with its range of movement the joint may react by forming a synovial *effusion*. Loose bodies most commonly affect the knee and elbow but they can occur in the hip, ankle and shoulder and will be visible on the radiographs provided they contain an ossified or calcified portion.

Causes of loose bodies in joints include:

(1) Osteoarthritis—separation of osteophytes.
(2) Osteochondritis dissecans.
(3) Fractures.

Neoplastic conditions

Tumours of the locomotor system fall into two groups:

(1) *Secondary or metastatic tumours*—usually deposited in bone. These are the commonest tumours of the skeleton.
(2) *Primary tumours*—both benign and malignant are rare (less than 0.3% of all malignant tumours diagnosed in the United States between 1969 and 1971 were of bone)[1]. About 20% of primary bone tumours are found in young people.

Radiographic examination is very important in the diagnosis of bone tumours. New growths can provoke radical changes in the radiographic appearance of bone. Some of these lesions are *osteolytic*—producing areas of rarefaction—or *osteoblastic*, where an increase in radiopacity will occur. Pathological fractures may feature in certain types and stages of bone tumour. Certain tumours inside the cranium and face may have an effect on surrounding bony structure; some of these may be found only in this area of the body and so will be considered with the indications for radiography of the skull and face. A diagnosis may sometimes be made on the basis of X-ray evidence alone; however, some tumours may not be visible until much bone has been destroyed. Plain radiography of the suspect areas can be augmented by tomography, arteriography and even xeroradiography.

Metastatic tumours

Bone is a common site for deposition of secondary tumours. These are usually of epithelial origin and the commonest primary sites are:

(1) Breast.
(2) Bronchus.
(3) Thyroid.
(4) Kidney.
(5) Prostate.

Metastases may be blood borne and can be deposited anywhere in the skeleton, particularly vertebrae, flat bones and proximal ends of femur and humerus. Breast metastases are common in ribs, thoracic vertebrae and clavicles but can ultimately invade the entire skeleton. Prostate metastases may reach the bone by venous spread and are common in limbs, sacral spine and pelvis.

Metastases usually occur late in the development of the primary disease and sometimes a pathological fracture from (for example) carcinoma of the bronchus may be the first sign of the disease. Most secondary deposits are osteolytic but metastases from the prostate and very rarely from the breast are osteoblastic.

Primary neoplasms of bone tissue

Bones are made up of many types of tissue—bone, cartilage, fibrous tissue, marrow, etc.—and tumours can arise from most of these tissues as well as from associated soft tissues—muscle, fat, synovium, blood vessels, etc.—although soft-tissue tumours are comparatively rare.

A simple classification is given in *Table 3.1*; note that definite classification of primary tumours is difficult

Table 3.1 Classification of primary neoplasms of bone

Tissue	Benign	Malignant
Bone	Osteoma	Osteosarcoma
Cartilage	Chondroma	Chondrosarcoma
	Osteochondroma	
Marrow		Ewing's tumour, myelomatosis
Uncertain origin	Giant cell tumour	Giant cell tumour

because precise tissue of origin is often uncertain, mixed cell tumours are common and different areas of a tumour may contain different types of tissue.

Osteomas

These are usually benign. An *ivory osteoma* occurs mainly on the flat bones of the skull and is very dense and hard. A *cancellous osteoma* consists of slender outgrowths of bone with a cartilaginous cap and usually arises in the metaphyseal region near a joint—it is also known as an *exostosis* or *osteochondroma*. These may be solitary or multiple.

Osteosarcomas (Figure 3.12)

About one-fifth of malignant bone tumours are osteosarcomas. The tumour arises from the metaphysis of long bones and is usually found in the lower end of the femur, it is highly malignant and may metastasize to the lungs. Osteosarcoma tends to occur in individuals between the ages of 16 and 25. Patients over 65 with Paget's disease may develop an osteosarcoma, and a sarcoma may be induced by radiation.

Chondromas

These are benign tumours composed of cartilage cells found within a bone, most commonly in the finger bones of the hand.

Chondrosarcoma

Frequency of this tumour is about half that of osteosarcoma but on the whole rather less malignant. The tumour arises either from the ends of the major long bones or from flat bones such as the pelvis or scapula. A chondroma in a major long bone may undergo malignant change to become a chondrosarcoma.

Myelomatosis

Myelomatosis or multiple myeloma is a neoplastic proliferation of plasma cells or their precursors, usually confined to the bone marrow and occurring in elderly subjects. The

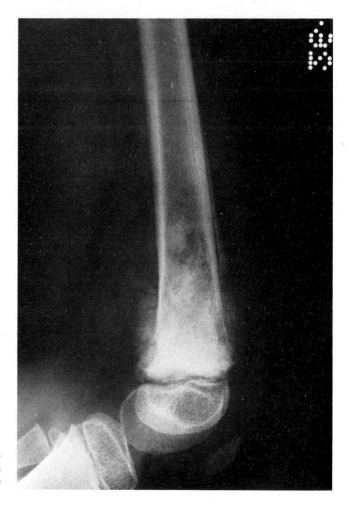

Figure 3.12. Osteogenic sarcoma in the left lower femur. On the anterior aspect of the bone the periosteum is raised abd new bone is seen to be forming underneath it

disease is often characterized by multiple foci of bone destruction. These foci appear as small 'punched out' areas involving the 'marrow bones' (long bones of limbs, skull, sternum, pelvis and spine) (*see Figure 1.6*).

Ewing's tumour

This is a highly malignant tumour affecting young people, most commonly between the ages of 5 and 20. The origin has not yet been completely clarified but most authorities accept that it arises from the endothelium of the bone marrow spaces. The shafts of femur, tibia and humerus are most commonly affected but it can also be seen in flat bones such as pelvis or ribs. Ewing's tumour metastasizes early and widely to lungs, lymph nodes and skull, and sometimes to the spine, scapula and clavicle.

Giant cell tumours

The origin of this tumour has been the subject of controversy for years. Another name for the giant cell tumour is *osteoclastoma* because it was once believed that the tumour arose from the osteoclast. The tumour may be either benign or malignant in which case it may metastasize to the lungs. It occurs in the ends of the long bones, usually the lower femur, radius or upper tibia and humerus.

Bone cysts

Bone cysts are tumour-like lesions which produce cyst-like cavities with thin bony walls usually found in long bones.

Soft-tissue neoplasma (*Table 3.2*)

Serious neoplastic disease is less common in soft tissues of the locomotor system than in bone. They may or may not cause changes in the radiographic appearances of bone. Visibility depends on the tumour's association with proximal or surrounding bone.

If it lies in muscle or fat its physical density may be sufficiently different to render it apparent; thus a tumour of high fat content may be visible because it is more radiolucent. Some soft-tissue tumours may be calcified.

Table 3.2   Soft-tissue neoplasma

Tissue	Benign	Malignant
Fat	Lipoma	Liposarcoma
Musculo-tendinous	Rhabdomyoma	Rhabdomyosarcoma
Synovial	Synovioma	Synovial sarcoma
Nervous	Neurolemma	
	Neurofibroma	Neurofibrosarcoma
	Neurofibromatosis	
Blood	Haemangioma	Haemangiosarcoma

Lipoma

Lipomas are common tumours occurring anywhere in the body where fatty tissue is present. They are easily recognized on radiographs by their lucent nature.

Liposarcoma

Very rarely malignant changes take place in liposarcoma.

Rhabdomyosarcoma

True tumours of muscles and tendons are rare. Very occasionally a malignant new growth of striped muscle occurs. A rhabdomyosarcoma is highly malignant and metastasizes rapidly.

Benign synovioma

These arise from the synovial tissue of joints and tendon sheaths, usually in the hand, and cause lobulated swelling.

Synovial sarcoma

This is a highly malignant growth arising from synovial tissue, usually of a major joint such as the knee. It metastasizes to the lungs.

Neurilemmoma

This is an encapsulated, slowly growing tumour which arises from the neural sheath and consists mainly of Schwann cells.

Neurofibroma

Neurofibromas arise from the fibrous tissue lining of a peripheral nerve and sometimes become malignant.

Neurofibromatosis

This causes multiple neurofibromas. It is hereditary and is associated with severe kyphoscoliosis and is one of the many causes of club foot.

Haemangiomas

These are probably not true tumours but a local congenital anomaly of blood vessels. Haemangiomas are more commonly found in the vertebrae, affecting a single vertebral body—destruction of the bone may result in its eventual collapse. Large congenital haemangiomas are considered to be arteriovenous communications. They are more frequently found in the lower limb. Because they cause an increase in local blood flow they can accelerate epiphyseal growth, resulting in a discrepancy in limb length.

Reference

1. CUTLER, S.J. and YOUNG, J.L., JR (1975). Third National Cancer Survey: incidence data. *National Cancer Institute Monograph*, **41**, 1–454

4　The radiographic examination

Guidelines for radiography of bone

(1) The minimum number of films to be taken, with few exceptions, is *two*, taken in *two planes* preferably at right angles to each other. A lesion may be missed if only one film is taken.

(2) Supplementary projections or techniques may be needed, especially where subtle fractures or other pathology are to be demonstrated: for example, axial projection of the patella, macroradiographs of the scaphoid bone, obliques in the vertebral column and tomography to prove the existence and define the limits of a lesion.

(3) Serial examinations may be needed: for example, to show a bony injury that is not apparent at the initial examination as in fracture of the scaphoid, to show periodic changes in a pathological condition and to assess the outcome of a particular regimen of treatment.

(4) Radiographs of the other side of the body may be needed for comparison, especially in children to compare epiphyses.

Terminology used in radiographic technique

The aim of using correct terminology is to help systematize the description of projections.

Many of the words used are derived from anatomy but it is assumed that the reader will already be familiar with general anatomical terminology for description of the aspects and planes of the body, and for describing the relative movements of the limbs. Anatomical landmarks and planes for the head are described and illustrated in Chapter 10. Examples of the terms especially relevant to radiographic technique are listed below.

Terms for general patient position

Supine—Lying facing upwards.
Prone—Lying facing downwards.
Erect—Standing or sitting.

Terms for specific projections (views)

These are derived from the direction in which the X-ray beam passes through the subject.

Anteroposterior (A-P)—The posterior aspect of the subject faces the film.
Posteroanterior (P-A)—The anterior aspect of the subject faces the film.
Lateral (Lat)—One side of the body or limb is next to the film. For the trunk and head, the median saggital plane lies parallel to the film. For the limbs a lateral projection can also be described as *mediolateral* or *lateromedial* depending on the aspect of the limb nearest the film.
Oblique—The trunk, head or limb is placed in a position that lies *between* the A-P or P-A and the lateral position.

In radiography of the head, alternative terminology may be used which has been derived from the names given to local anatomical areas or aspects of the skull. Examples are as follows:

Occipitofrontal (O-F)—The X-ray beam is directed via the occipital aspect of the head towards the frontal bone.
Occipitomental (O-M)—The X-ray beam is directed through the occipital aspect of the head towards the patient's chin.

Terms used to describe the direction of the X-ray beam

Cephalad or cranial angle—Rotating the X-ray beam through a number of degrees from a position where it is perpendicular to the film ('straight'), towards the patient's head.
Caudad or caudal angle—Rotating the X-ray beam through a number of degrees from a position where it is perpendicular to the film ('straight'), towards the patient's feet.
Unless the X-ray tube or beam angle is specified, the direction of the central ray is always taken to be perpendicular to the film cassette.

Immobilization of the patient

This is an important aspect of radiographic technique. Many repeat radiographs have been necessitated because of the movement of a badly immobilized patient.

The radiographer should appreciate how difficult it is even for the co-operative patient to maintain a position. Every reasonable step should be taken to ensure that the patient can remain still without undue discomfort.

Attempts at immobilizing the subject for the exposure start with the simple use of correct patient posture. He should lie rather than sit, sit rather than stand—as appropriate for each body part.

The resting of a limb or body part against the support is vital. For the upper limb up to the shoulder region in most techniques the *whole* arm should lie on the table top. When examining the lower limb if the patient is seated on the table ideally he should lean against a back rest. Any ploy to increase patient comfort helps him to keep still. Special but simple immobilizing devices should be freely available for *use* in every X-ray room. These include sandbags, non-opaque pads and bucky bands.

Protection of the patient from radiation

Radiographing a person inevitably involves irradiating him. Steps to reduce the dose include:

(1) Checking the patient's identity—examining the correct patient and undertaking the correct examination.
(2) Implementation of the 'ten-day rule' for women of childbearing age where possible. This rule is disregarded in an emergency where the benefit from the X-ray examination outweighs the risk associated with irradiating a woman who may be in early pregnancy.
(3) Getting the technique right first time—avoid repeat radiographs for whatever reason.
(4) Use of fastest film/intensifying screen combinations compatible with adequate image quality.
(5) Limiting the size of the X-ray beam. This has the additional benefit of increasing radiographic contrast because by reducing the volume of tissue irradiated less scattered radiation is produced and thus less reaches the film.
(6) Using lead protection over sensitive areas—the lower abdomen and upper thighs for gonads, in some instances the eyes for protection of the lens.
(7) Observation of the Code of Practice rules for radiographic equipment, e.g. X-ray tube filter and housing specifications.

Use of anatomical markers

A marker indicating the correct anatomical side (left or right) of the patient should be *irradiated* on the film during the exposure. The presence of the marker should be checked, preferably more than once along with the patient identification data.

The radiographic image forming factors—a summary

The radiographic technique and the image it produces is a system of recording information. The radiographer has two objectives:

(1) To select the appropriate projections for an area of the body and particular pathological condition.
(2) To produce images which have such qualities that the viewer can observe and detect the information they carry.

Assuming that the criteria for (1) are satisfied the image must then have three important qualities:

(1) It must have sufficient blackening (photographic density).
(2) The differences between the densities should be apparent (radiographic contrast).
(3) The amount of information per unit area should be optimal and appropriate for the subject being radiographed (detail and resolution).

Of course, this information is useless unless the viewer's brain can recognize it and interpret it.

The radiographer must be able to understand and thus manipulate the factors that can affect the radiographic image. The following is a summary of these factors.

Photographic density (film blackening)

The degree of film blackening achieved by the radiographic exposure and subsequent film development generally depends upon the amount of radiation (X-rays and light produced by the intensifying screens) that has reached the film.

For a particular subject, film blackening depends on:

(1) *The milliampere seconds* (mAs) selected. Increasing the mA increases the intensity of the X-ray beam. Increasing the exposure time lengthens the duration of the exposure.

(2) *The kilovoltage* (kVp) selected. The intensity of the beam increases as the kVp increases. The beam is also more likely to reach the film because it has greater penetrating power.

For a given radiographic exposure (mAs and kVp) and film emulsion type, the film blackening of the resultant radiograph is also determined by:

(3) *The size, physical density and atomic number of the subject.* Absorption of the X-ray beam tends to bear a proportional relationship to these characteristics.
(4) *The development process.* This is usually standardized throughout the X-ray department.
(5) The *type of intensifying screens* used with the film, e.g. 'high-speed' screens produce more film blackening for a given radiographic exposure than 'slow-speed' (detail or high-resolution) screens.

Radiographic contrast

The radiographic image is produced because some areas of the subject absorbs fewer X-rays than others. This results in corresponding areas of film receiving more exposure—thus becoming blacker after development.

If there were no changes in the level of photographic density over the whole radiograph then there would be no useful image. That is an extreme example. Differences in photographic density must be present, i.e. the film must have *radiographic contrast* so that an image can be seen.

Where the level of density difference is great the image is said to have *high contrast*. If very little difference is present then the radiograph has *low contrast*.

Radiographers and radiologists refer to the *optimum contrast* required in a radiograph, rather than simply stating that 'good' contrast should be achieved. This is because too much contrast can result in loss of information from the radiograph whilst too little means that information may be difficult to perceive. The level of contrast found acceptable by radiologists can vary.

Radiographic contrast depends on the following:

(1) *The subject* to be radiographed, e.g. bone absorbs a relatively large amount of X-rays because of its physical density and relatively high atomic number compared with soft tissue which is mainly water and has low density and atomic number. On most radiographs the bones are easily seen—they look 'white' when juxtaposed with soft tissue which is either 'black' or 'grey'. Thus a radiographic subject containing bone and soft tissue is said to have high *subject contrast*. Subject contrast can be altered by the use of *radiographic contrast agents*.

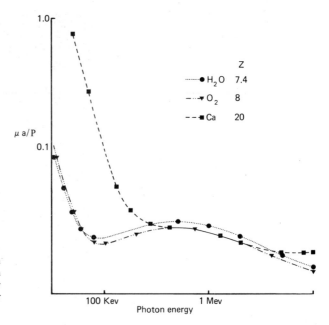

Figure 4.1. Variance of the mass absorption coefficients ($\mu a/\rho$) for water (soft tissue), oxygen (air) and calcium (bone) as the energy of the X-ray beam increases. The Z number (atomic number) for each substance is also indicated

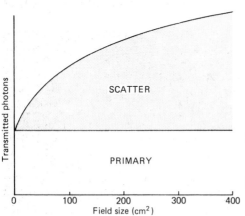

Figure 4.2. Ratio of scattered radiation to primary radiation transmitted by the subject for a given exposure but with increasing field size

(2) *The differences in the amounts of radiation reaching the film.* This is called *radiation contrast* and is obviously influenced by the subject. If a radiograph is taken only of soft tissue, the X-ray beam passing through the subject will not be changed very much. Where bone lies in the path of the beam, more radiation is absorbed and hence prevented from reaching the film. The mechanism of X-ray beam absorption varies at different photon energies (*Figure 4.1*). The differential in beam absorption/attenuation between soft tissues and bone decreases as kilovoltage increases. This principle is exploited in *high-kilovoltage technique* (*see* page 51).

(3) *Photographic factors* such as film type, development characteristics and the use of intensifying screens that enhance radiographic contrast.

(4) (i) *Amount of scattered radiation (Figure 4.2).* This can be decreased by reducing the volume of tissue irradiated—with beam collimators, cones, aperture diaphragms and compression devices. (ii) *Amount reaching the film.* This can be decreased with secondary radiation (scatter) grids or an *air-gap technique*.

Information content

Resolution means the ability of the recording system (film and its intensifying screens) to record fine detail.

Detail implies high information content on the film. The degree of detail recorded on the film depends on the resolving power of the film/screen combination. Resolving power is a numerical statement of resolution and is the

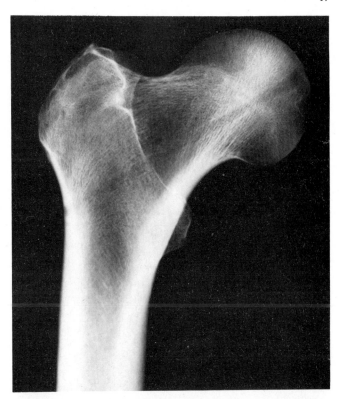

Figure 4.3. Radiograph of the upper extremity of the femur taken with 'high-resolution' intensifying screens. Compare with *Figure 4.4*

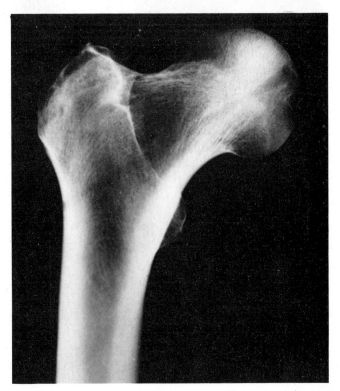

Figure 4.4. Radiograph of the upper extremity of the femur taken with 'fast' intensifying screens. Compare with *Figure 4.3*. The trabeculae appear to be less sharp or less detailed than in *Figure 4.3*

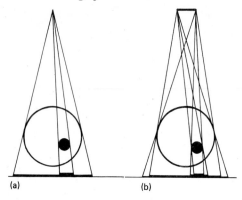

(a)   (b)

Figure 4.5. (a) Diagram of a radiograph being taken of an object using a theoretical point source of X-rays. There is no blurring at the edges of the object. **(b)** The same object is radiographed using a source of finite size. There is now blurring or 'penumbra' formation at the edges of the object. The size of the penumbra can be reduced by increasing the distance between the object and the source or the object and the film, and also by reducing the X-ray source size

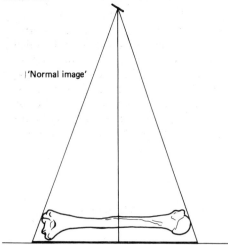

| 'Normal image'

Figure 4.6. Production of a 'normal' image

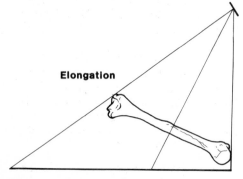

Elongation

Figure 4.7. Production of an elongated image

number of pairs of black and clear lines that can be recorded per unit length of the X-ray film when a test object is radiographed.

Most radiographs are taken using X-ray cassettes containing a duplitized film sandwiched between intensifying screens. Where *high resolution* is required in a radiograph in order to record a maximal amount of fine detail the appropriate screen/film combination is chosen. The disadvantage of using high-resolution screens is that they lack recording speed, i.e. a larger exposure will be needed to produce the correct film blackening and hence a larger dose of radiation is received by the patient (*Figure 4.3*).

If short exposure times are needed or if radiation dose should be kept to a minimum then high-speed screens are chosen. It is a general rule that where recording system speed increases resolution decreases (*Figure 4.4*).

The information content of the radiographic image can be reduced because of other factors. Blurring of the image is chiefly caused by *movement of the patient* during the exposure. *Geometric factors* also play a part because the source of the X-ray beam is of finite size (*Figure 4.5*). *Distortion* is a deformity of the image. In most projections the subject is deliberately positioned so as to maintain a parallel relationship with the film and a perpendicular relationship with the X-ray beam (*Figure 4.6*). Alteration of these relationships can result in *elongation* (*Figure 4.7*) or *foreshortening* (*Figure 4.8*) of part or all of the image. (In some situations this effect may be deliberately sought.) For each projection a specific X-ray beam *centring point* is given. Generally, the central ray of the X-ray beam passes through or close to the centre of the subject. The aim is to reduce image distortion caused by the divergent beam.

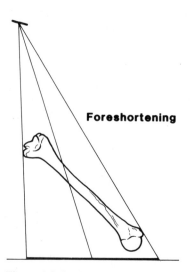

Foreshortening

Figure 4.8. Production of a foreshortened image

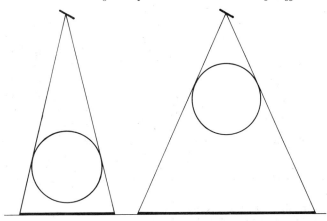

Figure 4.9. Magnification of the subject where the subject–film distance is large

Magnification is a type of image distortion although in some circumstances it may be deliberately introduced or tolerated. The X-ray tube focus-to-film distance (FFD) is fairly restricted because of the effects of the inverse square law which requires large increases in exposure as the FFD is increased. Standard FFD is usually between 90 and 110 cm. If a large subject-to-film distance is used, the diverging beam will project the X-ray shadow of the subject so that it covers a large area of the film, i.e. it will be magnified (*Figure 4.9*). The subject should normally be positioned as close to the film as possible. Where this cannot be done, in order to avoid a magnified image, the FFD should be increased thereby reducing the beam's degree of divergence. Magnification can be a problem in some X-ray tables where there is a large distance between the table top and film cassettes.

Consideration for the patient and other members of staff

Care and understanding of the needs and welfare of the patient during a radiographic examination should be high on the list of priorities for the radiographer. By adapting attitude and approach the radiographer should normally fulfil these requirements.

Out of the total number of patients referred for skeletal examinations, the majority will have come to the department because they have sustained some kind of injury. This may mean that many of the patients will have some difficulty in co-operating with the radiographer.

Whether or not there is trauma the radiographer should take into consideration the following:

(1) *The physical and mental condition of the patient.* This may be partially evident by the appearance of the patient. The

case history written on the request card may also help. The patient may need help in undertaking certain manoeuvres. Where pain or other pathological conditions are present gentle handling and modification of technique will be needed. Equipment designed to aid the examination of injured patients and others with limited mobility reduces the need for the patient to be moved or lifted.

(2) *The age of the patient*—whether the patient is elderly or very young. Special tactics and equipment have been devised to help deal with young children.

Other special situations for the radiographer are:

(1) *Radiography on the ward.* Take into account the patient's need for privacy and his need for comfort; do not place an uncovered cassette under the patient's bare back or bottom! Take extra care where there is equipment such as traction frames and wires, drips, oxygen and respirators in use. Ask permission of ward staff before going to X-ray the patient. Consider radiation protection for other patients and staff.

(2) *Radiography in an operating theatre.* Have everything you need ready, and check the equipment before the operation starts. This can minimize the time the patient spends under general anaesthetic. Use an aseptic technique where relevant. Consider radiation protection of other members of staff. Use a rapid film processing system to expedite the procedure.

(3) *Radiography of the seriously injured patient.* Speed and accuracy of technique is vital. Have everything to hand before you start, e.g. cassettes, grids, pads. Using special equipment such as the Siemens Orbix and an accident-table system such as the Siemens Koordinat Kombi will reduce the need for movement and handling of the patient. Blurring of the radiograph due to movement of the patient is more likely, therefore a faster film–screen combination must be selected to allow shorter exposure times. The patient may need holding—give an assistant radiation protection and adequate instructions. Take special care with badly injured limbs. When in doubt ask for advice and assistance from the medical and nursing staff.

Special radiographic examinations

Radiography undertaken with standard X-ray equipment and a film or film–screen combination is sometimes referred to as 'plain' radiography.

Special radiographic techniques are those that are supplementary or complementary to 'plain' radiography. These involve the use of special equipment and/or radiographic contrast agents and sometimes the manipulation of image-forming factors. In Part II reference will be made to these additional techniques but a detailed description of their application is outside the scope of this book.

Angiography—Radiographic examination where radiopaque contrast agent is injected into a vessel or duct. Angiography usually refers to blood vessels.

Arthrography—Radiographic examination where a contrast agent is injected into a synovial joint space for study of the soft-tissue structures. The contrast can be either a positive or negative type or sometimes both.

Arteriography—Synonym for angiography but refers especially to arteries.

Computerized tomography—A combined radiographic and electronic process which produces either transverse or longitudinal body sectional images. Information relating to X-ray absorption in the patient is processed by computer and presented visually on a television screen. Computerized tomography is not generally used for investigation of bone disease; however, it can sometimes be utilized where bony injury or pathology has also affected enclosed soft-tissue structures as in the skull, face, vertebral canal, thorax or pelvis.

Diffusion technique—The deliberate movement of part of the body so that overlying structures become blurred or diffused whilst the subject of interest remains relatively sharp. An example is the 'moving jaw' technique for demonstration of the upper cervical vertebrae in the anteroposterior plane.

Discography—Radiographic examination of an intervertebral disc by introducing a water-soluble contrast agent into the nucleus pulposus via a needle. Usually, more than one disc is examined.

High-kilovoltage technique—The equalizing of relative absorption of the X-ray beam by different types of tissue when a high kilovoltage is chosen. This technique is used for body areas where there is a steep difference in subject density, e.g. the cervicothoracic spine. High kilovoltage refers to kVs above 100. A major advantage is that a substantial reduction in mAs is possible. Because scattered radiation produced has greater energy it is more likely to reach the film. Either a high ratio grid must be used or an *air-gap* technique employed. In this technique a space is left between patient and film—the intervening air absorbs some of the scattered rays.

Macroradiography—A large subject–film distance is used which produces magnification of the subject. For a ×2 magnification, the subject is placed half-way between beam source and film.

$$\text{Degree of magnification} = \frac{\text{Focal–film distance}}{\text{Focus–subject distance}}$$

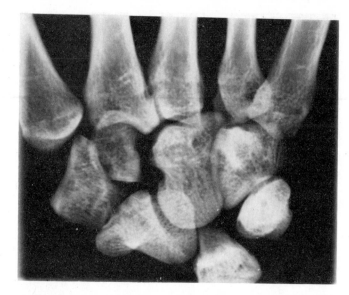

Figure 4.10. Macroradiograph of dry bones of the hand taken with a 'broad' focal spot (0.6 mm²). Compare with *Figure 4.11*

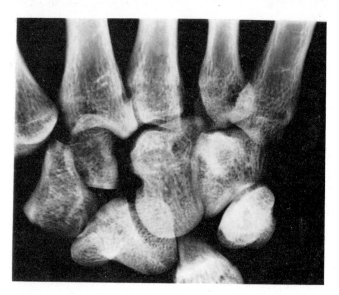

Figure 4.11. Macroradiograph of dry bones of the hand taken with a 'fine' focal spot (0.3 mm²). Compare with *Figure 4.10*

A very small focal spot size must be used in macroradiography otherwise geometric unsharpness, due to penumbra formation, will become very significant (*Figures 4.10* and *4.11*). Focal spot size should be about 0.3 mm².

Multiple (or steep-range) radiography—With a single exposure of the patient, several films are taken simultaneously. A range of tissue densities can be recorded when each film is exposed by intensifying screens of relatively faster or slower speed. A special cassette is used where the fastest film–screen combination is placed nearest the X-ray tube, and the slowest the furthest away. This technique is also known as '*steep-range*' radiography.

Myelography—The radiographic investigation of the spinal canal to demonstrate any obstruction to the passage of cerebrospinal fluid, e.g. a disc protrusion or tumour. The contrast agent can be either positive or negative.

Pneumoencephalography—The radiographic investigation of the ventricles of the brain following a lumbar puncture to introduce air into the subarachnoid space.

Radiculography—Radiographic examination of the spinal canal and nerve roots following introduction of water-soluble contrast agent into the subarachnoid space.

Radioisotope scintigraphy—This is not a radiographic technique but is an example of alternative imaging of the skeleton. Certain biologically active chemical substances can be injected into the patient's bloodstream and these are then taken up by bone tissue. If these substances, e.g. polyphosphonate or diphosphonate, are tagged with a radioactive isotope then this uptake may be recorded. Certain gamma-emitting radionuclides, e.g. technetium 99m, are suitable for this process and may be imaged by a gamma camera. The important difference between conventional radiography and scintigraphy is that where radiographs yield information about bone morphology and limited disclosure of bone physiology, scintigraphy produces a poor morphological image but considerable physiological (dynamic) data.

Scanography—Used in limb length measurements. A narrow beam of X-rays is moved down the whole length of the limb during a long exposure.

Tomography—The production of a radiograph of a selected *layer* in the body. All structures above and beneath this layer are blurred while the information contained in the layer of interest remain 'in focus'. Special equipment is required to undertake tomography. The X-ray tube and film cassette are rotated around a pivot point which coincides with the level required for the 'in focus' layer. The level of this pivot point can be raised or lowered thus producing consecutive radiographic 'cuts' (*tome*—Greek for cutting) in the subject. The rule is that the greater the degree of X-ray tube/film movement the greater the degree of blurring in the subject and thinner will appear the radiographic 'cut'. Tomography has extensive application in skeletal radiography. It is of special use in the skull and vertebral column where there is increased anatomical complexity.

Venography—Radiographic examination of the venous system where radiopaque contrast agent is injected into a vein. If this conventional venography is not possible because of occlusion or inaccessibility of the veins then the contrast agent can be introduced via a bone—*intraosseous venography*.

Ventriculography—The radiographic investigation of the brain ventricles following introduction of contrast agent via burr holes in the skull.

Xeroradiography—This technique uses conventional X-ray equipment in conjunction with special image-recording equipment. The range of X-ray intensities transmitted by the subject is recorded as an electrostatic charge density pattern on the surface of a special semi-conductor plate. This pattern of charges is then transferred to and made permanent on a piece of paper. The image is viewed by reflected light. Xeroradiography has been used to assist in fracture detection in the skeletal extremities and for demonstration of foreign bodies in soft tissue.

Part II

Regional radiography and pathology

5

The upper limb: hand to humerus

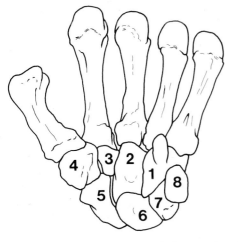

Figure 5.1. Anterior aspect of the carpal and metacarpal bones of the left hand

Indications for the X-ray examination

The hand

The skeleton of the hand is made up from three distinct types of small bone:

(1) More distally are the *phalanges*, the miniature long bones of the fingers. Each digit contains three phalanges except for the thumb which has two.
(2) The palm of the hand contains the five *metacarpals*, the thumb metacarpal articulating with the trapezium at the first carpometacarpal joint. This is a very mobile joint and probably the most important joint in the hand orthopaedically.
(3) Close to the wrist are the irregular or cuboidal *carpal bones* (carpus). The modern names for these bones are (*Figure 5.1*): 1, hamate; 2, capitate; 3, trapezoid; 4, trapezium (distal row); 5, scaphoid; 6, lunate; 7, triquetral; 8, pisiform (proximal row).

Injuries

Fractures of the phalanges

Various types of fracture occur. The casualty officer may strap the injured fingers together (*Figure 5.2*), so the radiographer may need to take posteroanterior, lateral and oblique views of the area of interest.

Mallet finger (baseball finger; Figure 5.3)

This is a deformity of the distal interphalangeal joint following an injury where the extensor tendon at the base of the distal phalanx is torn away from its point of insertion by

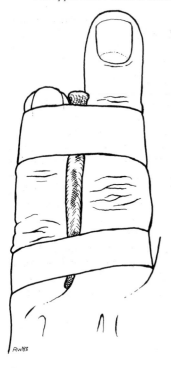

Figure 5.2. Strapping together of injured fingers

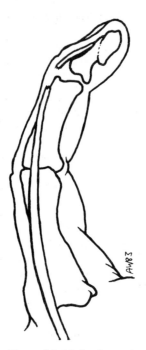

Figure 5.3. Mallet finger, showing the torn extensor tendon

a sudden flexion violence. Sometimes a small fragment of bone is avulsed by the tendon from the dorsal aspect of the terminal phalanx.

Dislocation of finger or thumb joints

Usually caused by forced hyperextension. A phalanx is displaced backwards at its joint with a more proximal phalanx or metacarpal. Occasionally the dislocation is associated with a vertical split in the joint capsule which becomes button-holed round the metacarpal neck making open reduction necessary.

Fracture of the neck of the fifth metacarpal (Figure 5.4)

This is a common injury usually sustained in blows made with a clenched fist. The head of the metacarpal is displaced anteriorly and the dorsum of the hand may appear to be deformed. Sometimes open reduction and internal fixation of the fracture are required.

Fracture of the base of the first metacarpal

The bone may be fractured transversely and the carpometa-

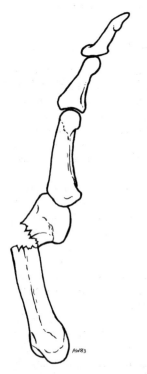

Figure 5.4. Anterior angulation of the head of the fifth metacarpal in a fracture of the neck

carpal joint is not involved. However, a more serious type of injury is sustained where the fracture extends into the joint.

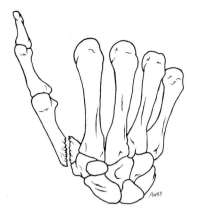

Figure 5.5. Bennett's fracture dislocation of the thumb metacarpal

This is known as *Bennett's* fracture dislocation of the carpometacarpal joint of the thumb.

Bennett's fracture dislocation (Figure 5.5)

In this injury a small triangular fragment of the first metacarpal remains in normal relationship to the trapezium whilst the rest of the metacarpal displaces proximally and backwards. If the surgeon cannot restore a smooth joint surface then the patient may develop osteoarthritis in this joint. Closed reduction is attempted first and the patient's forearm and hand will be enclosed in a plaster cast which is carefully moulded at the base of the metacarpal and includes the interphalangeal joint. The thumb metacarpal is held in extension at the carpometacarpal joint. The cast remains on for 4 weeks, during which time frequent X-rays through plaster are required to ensure that redisplacement does not occur. If closed reduction is unsatisfactory then the surgeon may have to resort to open reduction and internal fixation with Kirschner wires.

Fractures of the metacarpal shafts

If the fracture is of the transverse variety, there may be overlapping of the fragments with angular deformity.

Fracture of the waist or scaphoid (Figure 5.6)

This results from a forcible radial deviation of the carpus where the scaphoid is pinched between the radial styloid and the capitate. This fracture is most easily seen in the oblique radiograph of the wrist, but because of the nature of the scaphoid which has a very thin cortex and a cancellous medulla, there is sometimes no evidence of a fracture line on the initial radiograph. If clinical features have suggested that the scaphoid is indeed fractured but there is no radiological evidence then the wrist will be immobilized in a plaster cast and repeat films are taken 1 or 2 weeks later. If the scaphoid has been fractured it will almost certainly be seen at this stage because of bone resorption at the fracture line.

Complications in the healing of this fracture may occur because of the interference of the blood supply to the bone. Most of the blood supply to the scaphoid enters at its distal end. A fracture through the waist may cut off the circulation to the proximal fragment which may result in *avascular necrosis* (*see* Chapter 3). In time the shape of the scaphoid may become distorted and osteoarthritis could occur at the radiocarpal joint as a sequel. The diminished blood supply could alternatively cause *delayed union* of the fracture. Treatment of this may be by insertion of bone grafts.

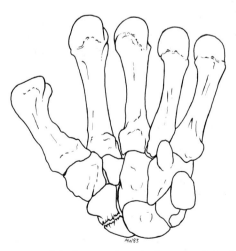

Figure 5.6. Fracture through the waist of the left carpal scaphoid

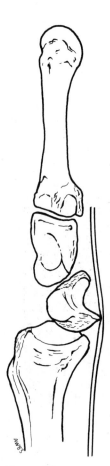

Figure 5.7. The lunate, dislocated from its normal position between the capitate and radius, impinging on the median nerve of the palm (sagittal aspect)

Old, ununited fractures of the scaphoid may sometimes be discovered by chance in patients who have radiographs taken of the wrist for some other reason.

Fractures of the lunate

These are relatively rare and result from acute dorsiflexion strains of the wrist. In the lateral projection a flake of bone can be seen on the dorsal aspect of the carpus.

Kienböck's disease

The lunate becomes flattened and sclerosed as a sequel to a minor injury (*see* Avascular necrosis, Chapter 3).

Dislocation of the lunate

Where an injury to the carpus involves forced dorsiflexion, occasionally the joint between the capitate and lunate becomes dislocated. As the wrist returns to the neutral position the lunate is displaced forwards and tipped through 90 degrees. This causes a characteristic change in the shape of the lunate as seen on the P-A film; it appears triangular instead of moon shaped.

The displaced lunate may now press on the median nerve causing paraesthesias (numbness and tingling) in the thumb, index and middle fingers (*Figure 5.7*). Avascular necrosis (*see* Chapter 3) in the lunate is a common sequel as the widespread capsular stripping may interfere with its blood supply. The surgeon may need to excise the lunate otherwise osteoarthritis may develop.

Other conditions

Carpal tunnel syndrome

This results from compression of the median nerve as it passes under the flexor retinaculum (transverse carpal ligament) of the wrist. This is a strong fibrous structure attached to the trapezium and scaphoid laterally and the hook of hamate and pisiform medially. The syndrome is common in middle-aged women but can occur in any situation where the volume of the tunnel is reduced, e.g. in a fracture of the lunate. Paraesthesias (numbness and tingling) in the thumb, index and middle finger are characteristic. Complete relief of symptoms usually follows operative division of the ligament.

Dupuytren's contracture

This is a thickening and contracture of the palmar aponeurosis and causes the fingers to be permanently flexed at the proximal interphalangeal and metacarpophalangeal joints. It is most common in the ring finger.

Osteoarthritis

Following an injury or rheumatoid disease, osteoarthritis may develop in the wrist joint. *Primary osteoarthritis*, however, (i.e. that which is not a sequel to other pathology) is more common in the carpometacarpal joint of the thumb (*see* Chapter 3).

Rheumatoid arthritis

Small joints of the fingers and the joints of the wrist are frequently the first to be affected by this disease (*see* Chapter 3). In the hand a characteristic sign of early rheumatoid arthritis is the appearance of juxta-articular erosions at the metacarpophalangeal joints (*Figure 5.8*). If the disease

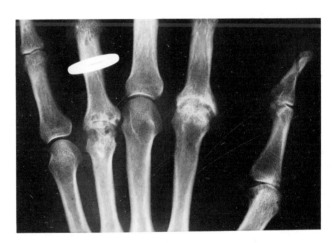

Figure 5.8. Radiograph showing changes in the fourth and second metacarpophalangeal joints characteristic of early rheumatoid arthritis

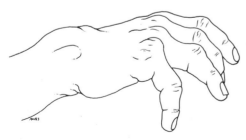

Figure 5.9. Deformity of the hand in advanced rheumatoid arthritis

progresses the fingers may take on a characteristic ulnar deviation at these joints, often associated with either flexion or extension deformities of the interphalangeal joints (*Figure 5.9*).

The wrist joint and forearm

The wrist joint lies between the lower end of the radius and the proximal row of carpal bones hence its name the radiocarpal joint. The lower end of the ulna is covered by a triangular cartilage so it does not directly take part in the wrist joint.

Between the upper and lower ends of the parallel radius and ulna are the radioulnar joints. Movement at these joints allows the radius to rotate around the axis of the ulna—the action of pronation and supination. This is the

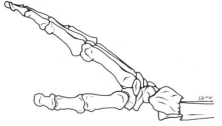

Figure 5.10. Colles' fracture of the right radius

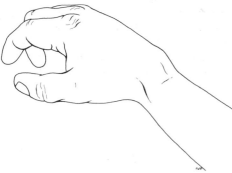

Figure 5.11. The 'dinner fork' deformity produced by the Colles' fracture

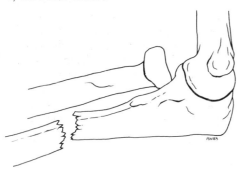

Figure 5.12. Monteggia fracture with anterior dislocation of the radial head

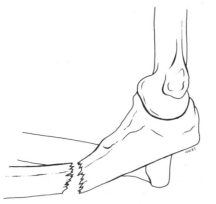

Figure 5.13. Monteggia fracture with posterior dislocation of the radial head

most significant function of the forearm and treatment of fractures must aim to maintain it.

Injuries

Wrist ligament and capsule strains

These are common sports injuries. If the patient has fallen on the outstretched hand the casualty officer may have to exclude a possible fracture in the region of the wrist.

Colles' fracture (Figure 5.10)

The radius is fractured within an inch of its lower articular surface. The ulna styloid is usually fractured as well. The distal fragment of the radius is displaced and angulated dorsally. The resultant characteristic appearance of the wrist has been dubbed the '*dinner fork*' deformity (*Figure 5.11*). The fracture is reduced under general anaesthetic and the wrist is immobilized in a 'below elbow' plaster.

Smith's fracture

Like the Colles' fracture this is confined to the distal inch of the radius but the displacement and angulation of the bone fragment is reversed—towards the palmar aspect of the wrist. This fracture is comparatively uncommon.

Forearm fractures

Fractures may be confined to one bone or may affect both. Where both bones are involved open reduction and internal fixation may be undertaken as the fractures are difficult to reduce and immobilize by external means. *Greenstick fractures* of the forearm are very common in children.

Monteggia's fracture

Fracture of the upper end of the ulna and dislocation of the superior radioulnar joint. Displacement may be either forward bowing of the ulnar shaft with anterior displacement of the radial head (*Figure 5.12*) or backward bowing of the ulnar shaft with posterior dislocation of the radial head (*Figure 5.13*). The injury often requires open reduction and internal fixation of the ulnar fracture.

Galeazzi fracture (Figure 5.14)

Fracture of the radius with dislocation of the lower radioulnar joint. The radial fracture may be internally fixed.

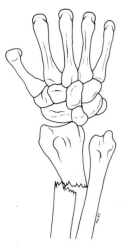

Figure 5.14. Galeazzi fracture

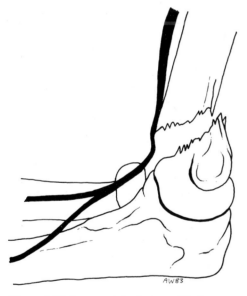

Figure 5.15. Supracondylar fracture of the humerus, the sharp upper fragment impinging on the brachial artery

The elbow

The elbow joint consists of two joints:

(1) A hinge joint between the trochlea of the humerus and the scoop-shaped trochlear notch of the ulna.
(2) A shallow ball and socket joint between the capitellum of the humerus and the head of the radius. Movement at the elbow joint is restricted to extension and flexion produced by the brachial (arm) muscles.

When the arm is extended at the elbow and lies in the anatomical position the long axis of the forearm is seen to make an angle with the long axis of the humerus. This is known as the 'carrying angle' and the wrist joint lies further away from the median plane of the body than the elbow joint.

Injuries

Supracondylar fractures of the humerus (Figure 5.15)

Common in children, usually caused by a fall on to the outstretched hand. (A similar force dislocates the elbow in an adult.) The fracture occurs in the lowest inch of the humerus and the lower fragment is usually displaced backwards. This fracture causes concern because there is a danger of damage to the brachial artery—ischaemia of the forearm is a serious complication. There is also a possibility of injury to the median and ulnar nerves. After reduction the elbow is held in flexion by the application of a collar and cuff sling. Some surgeons also protect the limb by means of a plaster-of-Paris back-slab.

Cubitus varus and valgus deformities

These are the result of excessive changes in the elbow 'carrying angle' due to mal-union of either a supracondylar fracture or some other fracture at the elbow.

Capitellum fractures

Commonly seen in children and young adults. In children diagnosis is difficult because of widely spaced centres of ossification. Closed reduction is impossible because the bone/cartilage fragment becomes displaced and rotated.

Olecranon process fracture

If the triceps undergoes sudden contraction and at the same time the elbow joint is forcibly flexed then the olecranon process (point of insertion for the triceps) may be snapped off the ulna and pulled posteriorly over the lower end of the humerus. This fracture requires internal fixation otherwise the hinge action of the elbow joint will be lost.

Coronoid process fracture

Seldom fractured except in association with a dislocation of the elbow. If this is the case the elbow may predispose to recurrent dislocation.

Fracture of the neck of the radius

This is a greenstick fracture characteristically seen in children following a fall on the outstretched hand.

Fractures of the head of the radius

This injury has the same causative force as a neck of radius fracture but characteristically occurs in adults. The fall drives the head of the radius against the capitellum. The fracture may only be a small vertical crack—hence supplementary projections are often required to demonstrate the injury. Alternatively the whole radial head may be comminuted in which case the surgeon may excise it as treatment. Sometimes the only effect of the fall is a bruising of the cartilage covering the articular surfaces but this is not evident on the radiograph.

Dislocated elbow

The elbow is normally a stable hinge joint, so if it becomes dislocated the joint capsule will be extensively torn. The ulna is displaced posteriorly or posterolaterally to the humerus and the radiohumeral joint is also dislocated. A characteristic sign of a dislocated elbow is the loss of normal alignment of the olecranon process relative to the epicondyles of the humerus.

After reduction under a general anaesthetic the elbow is rested in a collar and cuff sling. Although the joint is said to be stable to all forces after reduction the radiographer should nevertheless beware of attempting to extend the elbow for an A-P view. This may result in a recurrence of the dislocation!

Myositis ossificans

Ossification of muscle tissue, a rare but serious complication of a dislocated elbow.

Other conditions

Ulnar neuritis (elbow tunnel syndrome)

The ulnar nerve traverses a fibrous tunnel as it passes behind the medial epicondyle. Occasionally the sheath is too tight and the nerve is compressed. This gives rise to symptoms in the area of distribution of the ulnar nerve such as numbness or a tingling sensation (paraesthesias) over the ulnar border of the hand and the ring and little fingers, plus a weakness of the hand. Ulnar neuritis can also be a sequel to a fracture of the lower end of the humerus.

Osteoarthritis

In the elbow, arthritis may be a sequel to an injury that produces an incongruity of the joint surfaces. Osteophytes formed may break off and form loose bodies in the joint (*see* Chapter 3).

The humerus (lower two-thirds)

Fractures

These can occur at all levels of the bone and a spiral fracture may extend along the entire length of the bone shaft. A possible complication of a humeral shaft fracture is damage to the radial nerve which lies in the musculospiral groove.

The humerus is a common site for metastases from a carcinoma of the breast or bronchus, and often a pathological fracture is the first sign of abnormality.

Radiographic techniques

For the upper limb from the hand to the lower two-thirds of the humerus, most techniques can be undertaken with the patient sitting alongside the X-ray table. As much of the limb as possible should rest on the table top. A secondary radiation grid should not normally be required for the upper limb beneath shoulder level.

Hand

(1) Posteroanterior hand

The palmar aspect of the hand rests on the cassette. The fingers are separated slightly.

Centre—To the head of the third metacarpal with a vertical X-ray beam.

If both hands have to be examined, position them side by side on a single cassette.

Centre—Between the hands at the level of the head of the third metacarpal.

Individual fingers

Collimate the beam to include the distal phalanx and the metacarpal head.

Centre—To the proximal interphalangeal joint.

Injuries

The patient may not be able to extend the fingers and flatten the palm of the hand. It may be more practical to take an anteroposterior projection of the hand or individual finger.

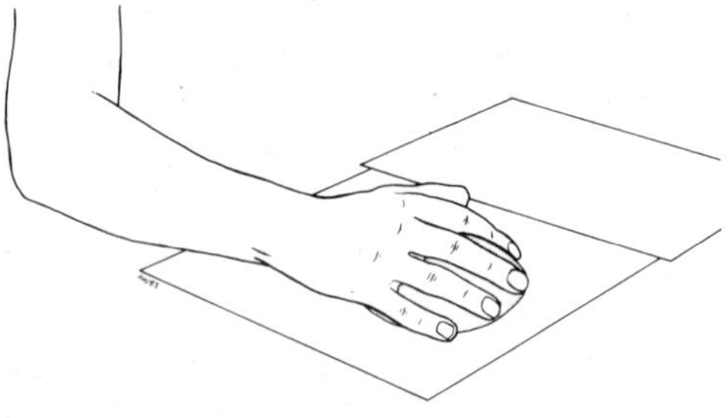

(2) *Posteroanterior oblique hand (Figure 5.16)*

With the hand pronated, the thumb side is raised until the palm makes an angle of 45 degrees with the cassette. The fingers and thumb are separated and flexed slightly.

The hand should be adequately supported on a non-opaque pad.

Centre—Over the head of the fifth metacarpal. Oblique rays produced by this eccentric centring point tend to reduce the overlapping of the metacarpals.

Figure 5.16. Position of the hand for the posteroanterior oblique radiograph

(3) *Lateral hand*

From the prone position, the hand and wrist are rotated laterally until the palmar aspect of the hand and fingers are perpendicular to the cassette.

Centre—Over the head of the second metacarpal.

The lateral can be used for location of a foreign body or to determine the degree of displacement of bone fragments in transverse fractures of the metacarpals.

Individual fingers

For the ring or little finger: use the last position. Fold forwards the index and ring fingers. Separate the ring and little fingers slightly; their long axes should be parallel to the film. The ring finger requires support.

Centre—Over the proximal interphalangeal joint of the appropriate finger.

For the index and middle finger: from the prone position the hand is rotated medially 90 degrees. The thumb, little and ring fingers are flexed palmwards out of the way of the index and middle fingers which remain straight but slightly separated. The lateral aspect of the index finger touches the cassette.

Centre—As above.

Where the proximal phalanx and the metacarpophalangeal joint is the area of interest, a posteroanterior oblique projection may also be necessary.

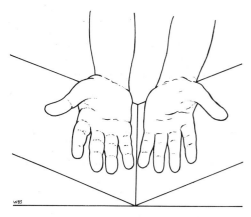

Figure 5.17. Position of the hands for Norgaard's projection

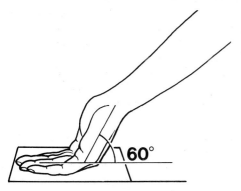

Figure 5.18. Position of the hand for Brewerton's projection

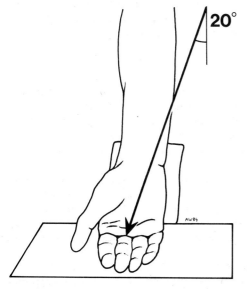

Figure 5.19. The X-ray tube angulation in Brewerton's projection

Rheumatoid arthritis

Two additional projections may be taken, as well as (1) and (2) cited above.

(4) Norgaard's projection (Figure 5.17)

Both hands are placed palms upward side by side on the cassette. They are both then rotated medially through 35 degrees and supported on non-opaque pads. The fingers and thumb are extended and separated slightly.

Centre—Between the hands at the level of the fifth metacarpal. The aim is to produce an image which avoids overlapping of the metacarpal heads and the bases of the proximal phalanges. This is an area where changes in the bone (erosions) caused by early rheumatoid arthritis may be seen but be obscured in the routine projections. The view has also been proved of value in indicating the presence of carpal erosions especially in the triquetral and pisiform.

(5) Brewerton's projection (Figure 5.18)

With the metacarpophalangeal joints of the affected hand flexed at 60 degrees and the thumb everted, the dorsal aspect of the fingers are placed on the cassette.

Centre—Towards the head of the third metacarpal with the X-ray tube angled 20 degrees from the vertical, from the ulnar side of the hand (*Figure 5.19*).

This demonstrates the grooves (valleculae) on either side of the metacarpal heads and also the bases of the phalanges. Erosions in the valleculae may be dubious or invisible in routine projections but may be shown to be large in this view.

Thumb

(6) Lateral

Starting with the hand prone, the fingers and the palm of the hand are raised slightly away from the cassette until the dorsum of the thumb is perpendicular to the film. Support the raised part of the hand on a non-opaque pad.

Centre—Over the first metacarpophalangeal joint to include the first metacarpal and trapezium.

(7) Anteroposterior projections of the thumb

Either (i) from the prone position medially rotate the hand and arm until the dorsum of the thumb lies on the cassette; or (ii) from the supine position laterally rotate the hand and arm until the dorsum of the thumb lies on the cassette.

Centre—In either case over the first metacarpophalangeal joint to include the first metacarpal and the trapezium.

In (i) soft tissues of the hypothenar eminence may obscure the trapezium and the carpometacarpal joint area. It may be easier if the patient sits with his back to the table and extends his arm behind him. (i) is easier than (ii).

(8) An alternative technique is to position the patient as for the lateral hand (projection (3)). Support the thumb, now in the posteroanterior position.

Centre—Over the first metacarpophalangeal joint as before for the thumb. Increase the focal–film distance by 10 cm to compensate for the increased subject–film distance.

Carpal bones

The distal end of the radius and ulna must be included on the film.

(9) Posteroanterior wrist

The palmar aspect of the wrist rests on the cassette. The finger joints are flexed slightly.

Centre—Between the radial and ulnar styloid processes.

(10) Lateral

From the posteroanterior position the wrist is rotated externally through 90 degrees. The ulnar aspect of the wrist and hand now rest on the cassette. An additional backward tilt is given to the wrist to superimpose the radius on the ulna.

Centre—To the radial styloid process. The carpal bones are superimposed in this projection.

If laterals of both wrists are needed for comparison the additional backward tilt can be omitted where both wrists are exposed simultaneously.

Centre—Between the wrists at the level of the styloid processes.

Laterals may also be taken in flexion and extension to demonstrate range of movement.

Techniques (11–16) are additional projections where further examination of individual bones is required.

(11) Scaphoid

(i) Posteroanterior with ulnar deviation

This is often used as an alternative to projection (9) rather than as a supplementary technique. The position is the same as in (9) except that the hand is adducted at the wrist as far as possible. The scaphoid can now be seen to be separated from the radius and its carpal neighbours.

(ii) Posteroanterior oblique wrist

From the prone position the hand and wrist are externally rotated through 45 degrees and supported.

Centre—To the ulnar styloid process.

This is an important view which reveals the waist of the scaphoid and its tuberosity which may more rarely be fractured.

Further posteroanterior oblique projections can be taken at angles of 30 and 60 degrees.

(iii) Anteroposterior oblique

The wrist is placed palm upwards on the cassette and then the radial side is raised through 45 degrees and supported.

Centre—To the ulnar styloid process.

(iv) Supplementary techniques

Because a hairline crack is difficult to detect, *macroradiography* and *tomography* may be chosen as supplementary techniques. *Radioisotope scintigraphy* has also been used but the technique has not been widely applied (*see* Chapter 4).

(12) Lunate

Posteroanterior wrist projection (9), this time with radial deviation.

(13) Trapezium

Posteroanterior oblique wrist [projection (11 (ii))] with ulnar deviation. The trapezium is also demonstrated on views of the thumb.

(14) Triquetral

From the prone position the radial side of the wrist is raised and rotated through 60 degrees. The wrist joint is palmar-flexed through 45 degrees.

Centre—To the triquetral with a vertical beam.

(15) Pisiform

This is demonstrated separate from the other carpal bones on the anteroposterior oblique of the wrist [projection (11 (iii))].

(16) Carpal tunnel

This axial projection demonstrates bony changes causing reduction of tunnel volume resulting in the carpal tunnel syndrome. The wrist is dorsi-flexed from the anatomical

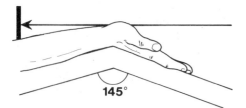

Figure 5.20. Dorsiflexion of the wrist in the axial projection of the carpal tunnel

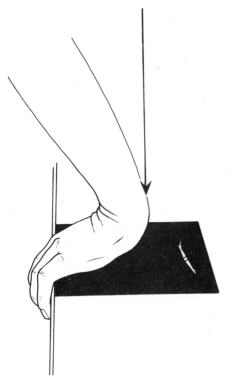

Figure 5.21. Alternative patient positioning for the axial projection of the carpal tunnel

position through 35 degrees. A special angle board can be used to achieve this (*Figure 5.20*).

Centre—Tangentially to the anterior aspect of the wrist so that the X-ray beam passes axially along the carpal tunnel.

An increase in the focal–film distance is necessary to offset effects of the large subject–film distance. Alternatively the wrist can be dorsi-flexed over the edge of the table (*Figure 5.21*).

Wrist (lower radius and ulna)

Two views are taken at right angles—a posteroanterior and lateral of the wrist including the carpus and the lower third of the radius and ulna.

Where injury to the forearm bones is not obvious a posteroanterior oblique wrist [projection (11 (ii))] should be included in case of fracture of the scaphoid. If injury precludes or limits the patient's movement then a horizontal X-ray beam may be used to produce the second view.

(17) Radiocarpal joint

This is a supplementary technique which aims to demonstrate the joint space. Position as for projection (9).

Centre—Midway between the styloid processes. The X-ray tube is angled 25–30 degrees towards the elbow joint.

Forearm

(18) Anteroposterior forearm

This demonstrates the whole length of the forearm bones. The forearm is raised on to the table and externally rotated until the posterior surface of the limb rests on the cassette. The styloid processes of the wrist are equidistant from the film. If possible the elbow is fully extended. Place a sandbag over the fingers.

Centre—To the middle of the forearm.

Producing this position may be difficult for the injured patient. A posteroanterior position is acceptable; however, the upper radius and ulna now overlap.

(19) Lateral forearm

With the forearm pronated the radial side is raised and rotated through 90 degrees until the dorsal aspect of the forearm is perpendicular to the film. The elbow remains flexed throughout. The hand should be immobilized.

Centre—To the middle of the forearm.

Wrist and elbow joints should be included on both projections. After the initial examination when the site of the injury is known it may be permissible to include only the joint nearest the injury on subsequent films. If the patient cannot rotate his arm because of injury then the two projections may be taken at right angles to each other using a horizontal X-ray beam for the second projection.

Patients in a long arm plaster

The position of the elbow and forearm is often such that the patient can't readily be placed in the posteroanterior or lateral position. Compensatory angulation of the X-ray beam may be required to produce satisfactory results.

Elbow

(20) Lateral elbow

The elbow is flexed to 90 degrees if possible and the arm is raised on to the table. The medial aspect of the elbow rests on the cassette. The wrist, elbow and shoulder should be in the same horizontal plane—use a table with adjustable height if possible. The forearm is rotated laterally until its dorsal surface lies perpendicular to the film. If this is not possible then a lateral elbow taken with the palm facing downwards is acceptable.

Centre—To the lateral epicondyle of the humerus.

(21) Alternative technique—For the patient with limited shoulder and arm movement. Leave the patient's arm in the sling and do not try to move it. The cassette can be placed directly behind the medial aspect of the elbow, resting between arm and the body (*Figure 5.22*).

Centre—To the lateral epicondyle of the humerus with a horizontal or suitably angled X-ray beam.

The patient remains seated or lying so the cassette should be adequately supported against the trunk. Radiation protection must be used. Place lead rubber between the patient and the cassette and collimate the beam.

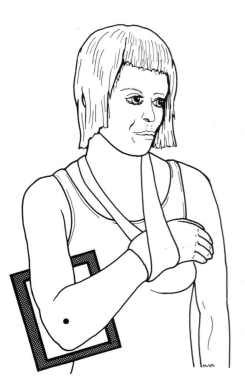

Figure 5.22. Position of the patient and film cassette for projection (21)

(22) Anteroposterior elbow

The whole arm is placed on the table with the palm and anterior aspect of the elbow facing upwards. The shoulder, elbow and wrist should all be in the same horizontal plane. The posterior aspect of the elbow lies on the cassette. Immobilize the forearm.

Centre—2.5 cm below the mid-point between the epicondyles.

Modified and alternative techniques—projections (23–25).

(23) For the patient who cannot straighten the arm fully, the elbow remaining slightly flexed

Choose one or more of the following three techniques according to the area of interest.

(i) The patient extends the arm at the elbow as far as possible and then places the forearm down on the table. Support the upper arm. The image of the humerus will be distorted according to how great its separation from the cassette. Increase the exposure by 5 kVp. *Centre:* 2.5 cm below the mid-point of the epicondyles.

(ii) Extend the elbow as far as possible except this time place the upper arm down on the table. Support the forearm. The distortion now occurs in the image of the radius and ulna. Increase the exposure by 5 kVp. *Centre:* Midway between the epicondyles.

(iii) Place the point of the elbow next to the cassette. Support both the upper and the lower arm. *Centre:* To the crease of the elbow. This produces equal amounts of distortion in the image of the humerus and radius and ulna.

Projection (24)

Often a patient may be able to raise the arm on to the table for the lateral view which is relatively easy but then cannot rotate the arm laterally for an anteroposterior view. After the lateral projection has been taken the arm remains in the same position. The elbow is raised slightly on a non-opaque pad. The X-ray tube is then turned through 90 degrees and directed so that the central ray is perpendicular to a cassette propped behind the point of the elbow.

Centre—To the crease of the elbow.

Projection (25)

For a patient with the arm fixed in extreme flexion because of injury or treatment immobilization, use either of the following:

(i) *Axial elbow, inferosuperior (Figure 5.23).* With the elbow in flexion the upper arm is placed in contact with the cassette. The palm is facing the shoulder.
Centre: Either 5 cm distal from the olecranon process with the X-ray tube vertical to show the olecranon process and the joint between the trochlear notch and trochlea of the humerus.
Or 5 cm distal from the olecranon process with the X-ray tube angled 30 degrees towards the shoulder to show the joint between the radial head and the capitellum.
Loss of image definition and increase in magnification

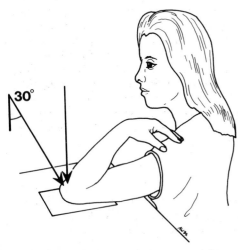

Figure 5.23. Position of the patient and directions of the central ray in projection (25(i))

must be expected in more distal parts of the radius and ulna.

(ii) *Axial elbow, superoinferior.* The patient sits with his back against the edge of the table. With the elbow flexed the arm is extended backwards over the table. The forearm is in contact with the cassette (*Figure 5.24*).
Centre: Just above the level of the humeral epicondyles with the X-ray tube vertical or angled towards the shoulder.

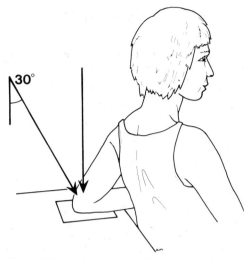

Figure 5.24. Position of the patient and directions of the central ray in projection (25(ii))

Patient on a stretcher

Where the arm is extended by the patient's side but cannot be moved, take two views at right angles using a vertical and then a horizontal X-ray beam. The arm is raised on a non-opaque pad. The X-ray tube may be angled to compensate for unsatisfactory patient position. Where the beam is directed at the patient's abdomen use lead rubber protection.

Children

Because the elbow has multiple centres of ossification comparative views of both elbows may be required.

Child with a supracondylar fracture

The patient may be seated in a chair or brought to the department on a stretcher. Do not attempt to extend the elbow joint. Do the lateral first using projection (21), for example. The anteroposterior view is taken in whatever degree of flexion happens to be present. The position of the forearm bones is largely irrelevant as what is needed is an anteroposterior view of the lower end of the humerus. If the elbow is flexed and the angle of flexion is extreme use projection (25 (i)). Where the elbow is in flexion but the angle is more than 90 degrees—do an anteroposterior view where the posterior aspect of the lower end of the humerus is in contact with the cassette, supporting the forearm. The child can be lying or sitting with the back of the arm against the cassette, placed for example in a chest stand.

Because of the scarcity of ossified cartilage, interpretation of the films may be difficult. Views of the other elbow may be requested for comparison.

(26) Head of radius

This can be visualized both on routine anteroposterior and on lateral projections (projections (22) and (20)).

Additional views for this area are as follows:

(i) From the true anteroposterior position of the elbow (projection (22)) the arm is laterally rotated to bring the head of the radius closer to the cassette. Some separation between the upper radius and the ulna is achieved. This position also demonstrates the proximal radioulnar joint. *Centre:* Over the head of the radius.

(ii) The anteroposterior position of the elbow with the forearm and the upper arm at 'equal-angles' [projection (23(iii))] gives an *'en-face'* view of the head of the radius.

(iii) When the forearm is pronated and supinated the ulna provides the axis of rotation and the radius moves round the ulna. Further lateral views of the elbow can be taken at stages of medial rotation—the radial head moving its position between each:
(a) Lateral elbow (projection (20)).
(b) Lateral elbow, palm facing down.
(c) Lateral elbow, forearm in full medial rotation.
(d) Lateral elbow with the beam angled 45 degrees up along the humeral axis.

(27) Olecranon process

This is demonstrated in the following:

(i) Anteroposterior elbow (projection (22)).
(ii) Lateral elbow (projection (20)).
(iii) Axial elbow, inferosuperior [projection (25(i))]. If the patient cannot flex the elbow to less than 90 degrees compensatory tube angulation towards the shoulder can be used.

(28) Coronoid process

This is demonstrated in the following:

(i) Anteroposterior elbow (projection (22)).
(ii) Lateral elbow (projection (20)).
(iii) From the anteroposterior position (projection (22)), medially rotate the arm raising the radial side through 45 degrees.
Centre: With a vertical X-ray beam over the coronoid process.

(29) Ulnar groove

A profile view. The position is the same as projection (25(ii)). The palm faces upwards and the elbow should be flexed at 45 degrees.

Centre—To the ulnar groove just lateral to the medial epicondyle. Use a vertical X-ray beam.

Humerus, lower third

An injury or pathology may involve the lower end of the bone. Two projections at right angles can be taken using similar techniques to that described for the elbow, if necessary increasing the area covered by the film.

Humerus, full length

It may be necessary to demonstrate the entire length of the bone including the shoulder and elbow joints.

(30) Anteroposterior humerus

The patient faces the X-ray tube. The arm is abducted slightly from the trunk, then supinated and fully extended at the elbow joint if possible. The patient is rotated slightly towards the side of interest so that the posterior aspect of the shoulder and elbow are in contact with the cassette or table.

Centre—Midway between the shoulder and elbow joints with a 'straight' X-ray tube.

The outer two-thirds of the clavicle and scapula should be included on the film. If the patient cannot fully extend the elbow, position him so that the posterior aspect of the upper arm is in contact with the cassette or vertical bucky. The mid-humeral centring point provides oblique rays which tend to project the forearm bones downwards. Where the elbow region is of special interest, further projections of that area should be taken.

(31) Lateral humerus

This is achieved by rotating the humerus medially 90 degrees from the anteroposterior position. The elbow is flexed and the arm is abducted and internally rotated. The medial aspect of the elbow should be in contact with the cassette or table.

Centre—Midway between the shoulder and elbow joint, with the X-ray beam perpendicular to the film.

This approach may be unsatisfactory because:

(i) There may be difficulty obtaining sufficient internal rotation of the arm.
(ii) It may not be possible to move the arm at all.
(iii) Rotation of the arm may not give a view of the humerus that is truly at 90 degrees to the anteroposterior projection.
(iv) The glenohumeral joint is still seen in the same plane as in the anteroposterior projection.

Alternative techniques—projections (32–34).

(32) If the patient can stand (Figure 5.25)

The patient faces the cassette or vertical bucky. The elbow is flexed and the forearm and hand rest on the abdomen.

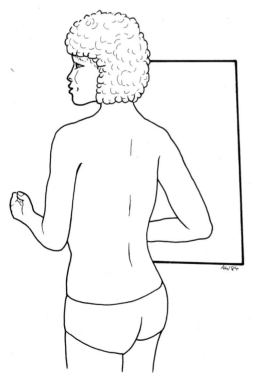

Figure 5.25. Position of the patient for projection (32)

The arm is abducted slightly from the trunk. Turn the patient's head away from the side under examination. Raise the uninjured side away from the film so that the lateral aspect of the elbow and the anterolateral aspect of the shoulder are in contact with the support.

Centre—Midway between the shoulder and the elbow joints.

The upper third of the humerus may be obscured by the bony or soft tissues of the scapular region and thus the exposure for this upper part of the arm may have to be increased. (Further alternative projections may have to be taken.)

(33) If the patient cannot move the arm at all

(i) *For lower two-thirds of humerus*—A cassette can be placed between the patient's arm and thorax. Lead protection can be placed between patient and cassette. (*See* projection (21).) *Centre:* to the lateral aspect of the elbow and humerus, perpendicular to the long axis of the bone with a horizontal or suitably angled X-ray beam.

(ii) *For upper two-thirds of humerus*—A cassette and grid are supported vertically against the lateral aspect of the shoulder. The opposite arm is raised over the patient's head separating the two heads of humerii. If the patient can stand, the positioning can take place against the vertical bucky—a grid should be used because of the large volume of body tissue the beam must traverse. The area covered in this projection may be extended by collimation to include most of the humerus but projections of the lower humerus via the abdomen should be avoided because of increased radiation dose to the patient. *Centre:* a horizontal X-ray beam is directed through the axilla of the raised arm towards the upper third of the humerus.

The exposure is made on arrested respiration.

(34) If the patient has limited movement and cannot raise the opposite arm (Figure 5.26)

A cassette is propped against the lateral aspect of the upper arm. The X-ray beam is directed transversely, separating the two sides.

Although not a true lateral it gives a second view of the humerus in the seriously injured or otherwise immobile patient. The upper extremity of the humerus will be obscured by the thorax.

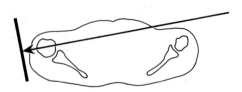

Figure 5.26. Position of the film cassette and the direction of the central ray in projection (34)

6   The shoulder girdle and thorax

Indications for the X-ray examination

The shoulder girdle

The bones of the shoulder girdle include the head of the humerus, the clavicle and the scapula.

The shoulder or glenohumeral joint is a 'ball and socket joint', the rounded head of the humerus articulating with the ellipsoid glenoid cavity of the scapula, a bony socket made deeper by its fibrocartilaginous rim, the glenoid labrum.

The outer aspect of the humeral head bears two bony prominences, the greater and lesser tuberosities, into which are inserted the tendons of the rotator cuff. These include the tendons of the supraspinatus, infraspinatus, teres minor and subscapularis muscles which blend with the capsule of the shoulder joint. The muscles of the cuff originate from the blade-like scapula.

The function of the clavicle is to act as a 'prop' for the shoulder joint, its lateral end forming a joint with the acromion of the scapula. Extra security is given to the position of the clavicle because of its attachment to the coracoid process of the scapula and the first rib by strong ligaments.

Injuries

Fracture of the surgical neck of humerus

This is often seen in elderly women. The degree to which the fracture fragments are displaced is variable and they are often firmly impacted so that the bone moves as one piece. In this instance the fracture may be overlooked (unless a radiograph is taken) because the patient may be able to use the arm to some extent without severe pain. Impaction is important because it will influence the surgeon's method of treatment. In children the injury that corresponds to a fracture of the surgical neck of the humerus is a *fracture separation of the epiphysis* from the upper end of the humerus.

Shoulder joint dislocation

The glenoid cavity of the scapula is shallow in order to allow a really wide range of movement at the shoulder joint—the joint depending for its stability on soft-tissue structures such as the long head of biceps, the joint capsule and the surrounding deltoid muscle. Dislocation is a very common injury in adults, usually caused by a fall on the outstretched arm.

There are three types:

(1) *Anterior dislocation (Figure 6.1)*—the humeral head is forced out of the glenoid cavity and comes to lie below the coracoid process. Because the greater tuberosity no longer holds out the deltoid muscle, which now falls as a curtain from the outer edges of the acromion, the normal curved contour of the shoulder is replaced by an acute angle or 'cut off' appearance (*Figure 6.2*).
(2) *Posterior dislocation*—relatively uncommon. The head of the humerus lies behind the glenoid cavity.
(3) *Inferior dislocation*—also rare. The head of the humerus lies beneath the glenoid cavity.

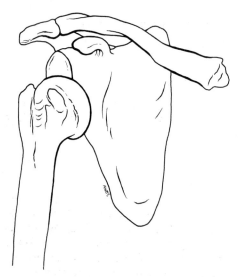

Figure 6.1. Anterior dislocation of the right shoulder joint

Recurrent anterior dislocation of the shoulder joint (Figure 6.3)

If the patient has a history of traumatic dislocation of the shoulder a situation may subsequently develop where the joint may repeatedly dislocate. This is usually due to the presence of an unhealed tear in the attachment of the glenoid labrum to the anterior margin of the glenoid cavity (*Bankart lesion*). This rent allows the capsule to balloon forward so that the humeral head can pass over the rim of

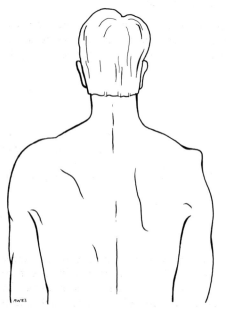

Figure 6.2. Appearance of an abnormal right shoulder in anterior dislocation

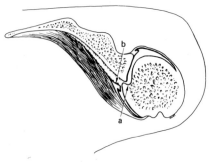

Figure 6.3. Transverse section through a left shoulder joint affected by recurrent anterior dislocation. (**a**) Notch formed on the head of the humerus. (**b**) Tear in the capsular attachment

the glenoid cavity. Recurrent dislocation can occur with a progressively smaller amount of force and after some time the joint becomes very lax and may dislocate on very mild external rotation of the shoulder, e.g. on opening a newspaper. Treatment of recurrent dislocation is by surgical repair. A notch may develop on the back of the humeral head or the anterior margin of the glenoid fossa where the bones undergo repeated contact each time the dislocation occurs.

Change in the shape of the humeral head in recurrent dislocation is sometimes referred to as the *hatchet deformity*.

Fractures of the greater tuberosity

These may be caused by a direct blow to the shoulder or may occur in association with dislocation of the shoulder joint.

Injuries of the rotator cuff

In a fall, if the abducted arm is forcefully brought to the side, the rotator cuff may be extensively torn. This usually involves mainly the supraspinatus tendon, which is normally subjected to the greatest mechanical strains. If the tendon is torn, the patient will be unable to initiate abduction of the shoulder—the action of the supraspinatus.

Rupture of the long head of biceps tendon

An injury of elderly patients often occurring spontaneously and associated with attrition of the tendon as it passes through the bicipital groove, the surface of which may be roughened.

Fractures of the scapula

These are caused by direct blows to the bone. They are uncommon, usually affecting either the neck or the body of the scapula. As the bone is an important site for muscular origins, the surgeon will be more concerned about soft tissue than bony injury.

Fractures of the clavicle

This bone is usually fractured at the junction of its middle and outer thirds. The lateral fragment is usually displaced downwards and medially. The fracture is reduced by applying traction along the line of the bone and this is achieved by 'bracing the shoulders back' with a special 'figure of eight' bandage.

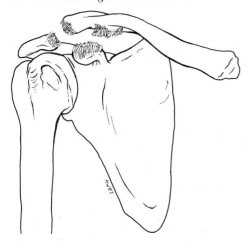

Figure 6.4. Dislocation of the acromioclavicular joint. Both joint capsule and coracoclavicular ligament are torn

Acromioclavicular joint injuries

Dislocation (*Figure 6.4*) is rare—subluxation is more common, resulting from a blow on the shoulder forcing the acromion downwards. The joint capsule will be torn but the joint cannot be displaced unless the strong coracoclavicular ligament has been torn.

Sternoclavicular joint injuries

The joint may rarely be dislocated, although fracture of the clavicle is far more likely. If the medial end of the affected clavicle is depressed it may impinge on the trachea and cause respiratory difficulties.

Other conditions

Rheumatoid arthritis

The shoulder joint is commonly affected in rheumatoid disease but usually in association with other joints. Tears of the rotator cuff occur more commonly in patients with rheumatoid disease.

The sternoclavicular joints can also become affected by rheumatoid arthritis (*see* Chapter 3). Destruction of the cartilage and the articular ends of the bones occurs in the same manner as in other joints.

Osteoarthritis

Osteoarthritis is rare because the shoulder is not a weight-bearing joint (*see* Chapter 3). If the patient is affected and also suffers from osteoarthritis in joints of the lower limb then this could be very disabling because he may not be able to make use of crutches. Osteoarthritic changes may sometimes occur in the acromioclavicular joints.

Calcific tendinitis

Calcification in the shoulder joint is most commonly due to calcific deposits within the tendons of the rotator cuff. The insertion of the supraspinatus is the most frequently involved.

Supraspinatus tendinitis

This inflammatory condition is usually localized to the upper part of the rotator cuff region of the capsule of the shoulder joint. The condition may progress to spontaneous rupture of the supraspinatus tendon. The radiographs may show calcification just above the greater tuberosity.

Frozen shoulder

This affects the middle aged and elderly. It is characterized by pain and stiffness in the shoulder joint—all shoulder movements are restricted.

Sprengel's shoulder

A rare congenital condition where the scapula is smaller and higher than normal (*see* Klippel–Feil syndrome, Chapter 8).

Craniocleidodysostosis (Figure 6.5)

This is a failure in the development of membrane bone in the skull, clavicle and pubic bones. The clavicles are either absent or the outer half of the bones are missing (*see* Chapter 10).

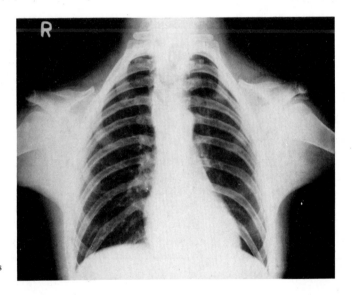

Figure 6.5. Craniocleidodysostosis—the clavicles are absent

The bony thorax

The walls of the bony thorax are made up of the ribs supported anteriorly by the sternum and articulating posteriorly with the dorsal vertebrae. The functions of the thorax are to protect its vulnerable contents and to assist in the provision of the respiratory movements. Separating the trunk from the abdomen is the diaphragm which is attached to the lower ribs and costal cartilages. During breathing the actions of the intercostal muscles and diaphragm produce alteration in the volume of the thorax. This is possible because the posterior end of each rib forms a pair of articulations with the dorsal vertebrae known as the costotransverse and costovertebral joints. Movement at these joints allows the rib cage to expand.

Injuries

Fractures of the ribs

Ribs are most frequently fractured as the consequence of compression of the thorax and this is most likely to occur during a road-traffic accident or fall. Ribs can bend under stress but if too much force is exerted then they will break. A fracture is usually located in the weakest area of the rib in front of the angle. In compression injuries the *middle ribs* are most commonly involved and rib fractures may be single, multiple, one-sided or bilateral and the fragments may or may not be displaced. Quite often rib fractures have no serious consequences for the patient—the ribs are largely splinted by the intercostal muscles—but where there is involvement of internal viscera then the injury is more serious. About half of traffic deaths result directly or indirectly from chest injury[1]. Note that intrathoracic damage may have occurred without bony injury to the walls of the chest (which includes the sternum and spine).

The following conditions may arise as a result of injury to the chest:

Pneumothorax—Lacerations of the pleura allow air into the pleural space and there is a collapse of underlying lung tissue which may vary in severity.

Haemothorax—Bleeding into the pleural space largely from lacerated intercostal vessels. If this bleeding is considerable then the patient may require a thoracotomy.

Traumatic emphysema (Figure 6.6)—Air enters the chest wall through a break in the pleura and distends the

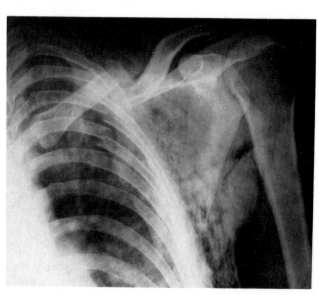

Figure 6.6. Radiograph of the left upper thorax and shoulder girdle showing rib fractures and traumatic emphysema. Note also the fractured clavicle

subcutaneous tissue. Tears in the pleura can be the result of either the rib fracture or be caused by the shearing force of the trauma.

Flail chest

Where there are several adjacent ribs fractured in two places or bilaterally. A *flail segment* is formed which is sucked in during inspiration and pushed out during expiration. This is known as paradoxical breathing and normal ventilation may be severely impaired.

Lower rib fractures

There may be associated injury to the diaphragm and upper abdominal organs, e.g. liver, kidney and spleen.

First and second rib fractures

These are relatively uncommon and may follow a severe downward blow which would also involve the clavicle. An isolated fracture of the first or second rib may be a *stress fracture*, caused for example by building-site hod carrying.

Sternal fractures

Comparatively rare and often the result of direct violence to the chest such as a steering-wheel injury. There is apparently a high mortality rate because violence severe enough to fracture the sternum may also cause serious intrathoracic injuries, e.g. rupture of the aorta.

Most fractures occur in the body of the sternum or near its junction with the manubrium, and they are frequently of the transverse type.

Other conditions

New growths

Metastases may occur in the ribs from a primary tumour in the breast (*see* Chapter 3). Ribs may also be destroyed by tumour infiltration from a lung carcinoma. New growths in the sternum are usually of a metastatic nature.

Other pathology of ribs

Ribs may be involved in any disease process of bone tissue, for example Paget's disease.

Evidence of previous thoracotomy

A rib may be displaced or become irregular, usually the 4th, 5th or 6th. This may be the only indication on the film that there has been surgery.

Rib notching

Indentations may be present on the inferior border of the posterior third of the ribs. The most frequent cause of this is *coarctation of the aortic arch* and the notching is due to dilatation of the intercostal arteries.

Congenital anomalies of ribs

The anterior end of a rib may be bifid or a rib may be absent. Ribs may articulate with or touch their neighbours. One or a pair of ribs may be present at the seventh cervical vertebra—*cervical rib* (*see* Chapter 8).

Abnormal curvatures of the spine such as *kyphosis* and *scoliosis* will affect the spacing and direction of the ribs. In kyphosis the posterior parts of the ribs are crowded together, in scoliosis the ribs are more vertically inclined on the concave part of the spine (*see* Chapter 8).

Congenital depressed sternum

This is a malformation that is not in itself an indication for radiography but the appearances of the posteroanterior chest radiograph are characteristic. The posterior ends of the ribs are horizontal, and the anterior ends slope down and inwards. The silhouette of the heart is altered due mainly to rotation about its vertical axis. The changes in the heart appearance may be misinterpreted as indicative of heart or lung disease.

Radiographic techniques

Shoulder

For radiography of the bones of the shoulder girdle a secondary radiation grid is considered to be optional except where the patient is significantly muscular and hence larger exposures are needed.

Direct exposure of a cassette for example in the anteroposterior shoulder projection tends to produce a 'grey' radiograph which is favoured by many radiographers because a wider range of subject densities becomes apparent. Using a grid technique frequently results in non-demonstration of the acromioclavicular area because it is superficial and easily over-exposed. A bucky grid is normally used for the lateral projection of the scapula.

(1) Anteroposterior shoulder

The patient faces the X-ray tube. If the patient is erect the elbow should be flexed and supported. If the patient is horizontal the arm is extended and abducted slightly if possible. Rotate the patient slightly towards the side under examination; the posterior aspect of the shoulder and humerus lies against the cassette or table.

Centre—To the head of the humerus. The film should include the outer two-thirds of the clavicle.

Children

An anteroposterior film of the other shoulder may be requested for comparison. Doubt may exist over the presence of bony injury in the head and neck of the humerus due to the normal appearance of the epiphysis and the epiphyseal line.

(2) Glenohumeral joint

In order to obtain a profile view of the glenoid cavity the patient must be rotated 45 degrees towards the affected side from the anteroposterior position (1). The arm should be abducted slightly and the elbow flexed, the hand resting on the abdomen.

Centre—To the head of the humerus.

The clavicle will be considerably foreshortened in this projection.

(3) Lateral shoulder

The patient should be able to abduct the arm at the shoulder joint for this projection.

The patient is seated alongside the table. Use either a curved cassette or an ordinary cassette placed in the axilla. The arm is extended over the cassette and the elbow is flexed for support. The neck is flexed and moved away from the side under examination (*Figure 6.7*).

Centre—From above towards the head of the humerus.

Difficulty may be experienced with this technique due to the following:

(i) Inability of the patient to extend the arm adequately.
(ii) It may not be possible to position the cassette far enough into the axilla to include the glenoid of the scapula on the film. Positioning of the cassette may be aided by placing a non-opaque pad underneath it. Angling the cassette slightly towards the thorax and angling the beam 10 degrees distally along the axis of the arm may help to solve these problems.

Alternative techniques—projections [(4(i)), (4(ii)) and (5)].

(4) Where the patient has limited movement

(i) A '*transthoracic lateral*' may be taken (*see* projection (33(ii)), page 76).

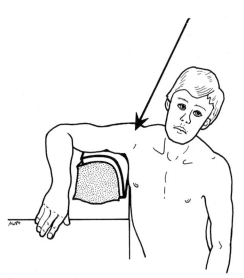

Figure 6.7. Position of the patient and curved film cassette for the lateral (axillary) shoulder projection

(ii) An *inferosuperior projection*. With the patient either recumbent or standing a cassette is placed above the shoulder joint and supported. The X-ray tube surface of the cassette faces the superior aspect of the shoulder. The arm is abducted to 90 degrees if possible.

Centre—From below the axilla towards the head of the humerus.

The degree of distortion of the upper humerus depends on the extent of arm abduction achieved by the patient.

Dislocation of the shoulder

If an *anterior dislocation* is present then it will be readily identified on the anteroposterior radiograph and certified by clinical examination. A *posterior dislocation (Figure 6.8)* is not so obvious and the anteroposterior radiograph may look 'normal'.

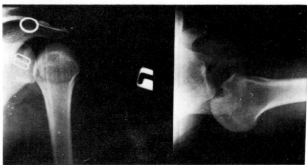

Figure 6.8. Anteroposterior and lateral (axillary) radiographs of the left shoulder. The patient has a posterior dislocation of the humeral head

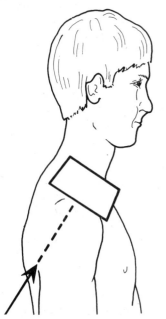

Figure 6.9. Film cassette position and direction of the central ray for projection (5)

As the patient may have difficulty in abducting the arm the transthoracic lateral projection (*see* projection 33(ii), page 76) may be the obvious choice of technique for a second projection. However, the relationship between the glenoid cavity and the head of the humerus may not be readily seen. If alternatives (3) or (4(ii)) cannot be done then the following modification should be used.

(5) (*Figure 6.9*) The patient can be seated or standing. The cassette is supported above the patient's shoulder (and can be held by the patient). The X-ray beam is directed from below the axilla and from *behind* the patient towards the shoulder joint. To avoid the trunk the X-ray tube can be angled forwards and the cassette angled appropriately to be perpendicular to the central ray.

Recurrent dislocation of the shoulder

Further anteroposterior and axillary projections of the shoulder [projections (1), (4(ii))] can be taken with the arm in varying degrees of internal and external rotation. The relationship between the humerus and glenoid cavity alters, revealing different aspects of the humeral head.

Special projections may be required to demonstrate the

notch or compression defect that forms on the back of the humeral head in some cases of recurrent anterior dislocation.

(6) (i) With the patient supine the arm is raised and the palm of the hand is plaed on top of the head. The arm is also rotated medially so the elbow faces in a forward direction. *Centre:* to the coracoid process with the X-ray tube angled 10 degrees cephalad.

(6) (ii) *Anteroposterior shoulder* (projection (1)). *Centre:* to the coracoid process with the X-ray tube angled 45 degrees caudad.

Further information may be sought with *arthrography*.

Calcification of rotator cuff tendon sheaths

The following are profile projections (7–11) of the regions of the tendinous insertions. It is sometimes difficult to localize precisely calcifications in *infraspinatus* and *teres minor* because of the high mobility of the shoulder joint. Lesions may also occur in the bone at the points of insertion. The patient should be recumbent to aid immobilization. Exposure technique should aim to demonstrate soft tissue as well as bony detail.

Again, further information may be sought with *arthrography*.

(7) Supraspinatus

Anteroposterior projections (1) with (7(i)) a 'straight' X-ray tube; or (7(ii)) the X-ray tube angled 30 degrees caudad; or both. The second projection demonstrates the space between acromion and head of humerus.

(8) Subscapularis

Anteroposterior projections (1) with (8(i)) the patient's arm supinated; and (8(ii)) in internal rotation; and (8(iii)) in external rotation.

If the calcification is in the subscapularis tendon it will appear to displace medially on internal rotation whereas calcification in the supraspinatus tendon will lie in a relatively constant position. A profile projection of the *bicipital groove* (11) shows the calcification towards the medial margin of the groove (insertion into the lesser tuberosity). An inferosuperior projection (4(ii)) with the arm abducted to 90 degrees demonstrates the calcification over the lesser tuberosity.

(9) Infraspinatus

Anteroposterior projection (1) with (9(i)) the patient's arm in external rotation and (9(ii)) the X-ray tube is angled 25 degrees caudad.

(10) Teres minor

Anteroposterior (1) with patient's arm in full internal rotation.

(11) Bicipital groove

This is a profile projection and is best done with the patient supine for immobilization. The arm lies in extension and is abducted about 20 degrees and rests on the couch by the patient's side. A cassette is propped vertically above the head of the humerus and the central ray has to be directed along the axis of the bicipital groove.

Centre—With the beam angled 10 degrees from the horizontal towards the long axis of the humerus to the anterior surface of the head of humerus and tip of the acromion.

Scapula

Exposures for the scapula should be made on arrested respiration; however, a *diffusion* exposure technique can be applied to the anteroposterior projection (*see* pages 51 and 93).

(12) Anteroposterior scapula

This can be taken with the patient supine but in cases of injury erect positioning may be easier. The patient faces the X-ray tube. Rotate the patient slightly towards the side under examination so that the body of the scapula is parallel to the film. The elbow of the affected side is flexed and the forearm is supported.

Centre—Over the head of the humerus. This centring point is lateral to the scapula and oblique rays project the ribs towards the vertebral border of the bone thus revealing a greater proportion of the scapular body.

The clavicle and upper third of the humerus should be included on the film.

Inferior angle of the scapula

Use projection (16(iii)) but in addition the affected side is raised slightly away from the film to separate the lateral border of the scapula from the rib cage.

Centre—Over the axilla.

(13) Lateral scapula

The aim is to produce a profile projection of the scapular body, superimposing it upon the neck, head and glenoid cavity. The head and possibly the upper one-third of the humerus will obscure part of the scapula in the lateral projection, the degree of obscuring will depend on how far the patient can flex or extend the arm at the shoulder joint thus moving the humeral shaft away from the scapula. The humeral head is inevitably superimposed on the glenoid cavity. Choose the following technique if the patient can co-operate fully.

The patient faces the vertical bucky. The head is turned away from the side under examination. The arm of the affected side is extended behind the body (by 40 degrees from the vertical), the elbow is flexed and the wrist rests on the iliac crest of the affected side. Raising the unaffected side away from the bucky the body is rotated through about 25 degrees (*Figure 6.10*).

Centre—Over the fourth thoracic vertebra.

The X-ray tube diaphragms are opened so that the oblique rays produced by this centring point result in a profile projection of the scapula. The cassette is off-centred towards the side under examination so that the scapula is centralized on the film (*Figure 6.11*).

Alternative techniques—projections (14) or (15).

Projection (14)

Where the patient has limited movement. The patient sits in the general lateral position where the median sagittal plane is parallel to the film. The shoulder under examination is nearest to the film. The arm of the injured side is placed across the trunk, if possible the hand of the injured side clasps the opposite shoulder. The side of the patient furthest from the film is rotated forwards through 20 degrees.

Centre—Over the vertebral border of the scapula at the level of the fourth thoracic vertebra.

Projection (15)

From the anteroposterior position (projection (12), patient sitting) the hand of the injured side clasps the opposite shoulder. The affected side is rotated forwards through 50–60 degrees until the scapula is seen in profile.

Centre—5–7.5 cm medial to the axillary border of the scapula.

The subject–film distance is notably increased therefore focal–film distance could be increased to offset magnification of the scapula.

(16) Coracoid process

This is demonstrated with the following projections:

(i) Lateral scapula (projections (13), (14)).
(ii) Axillary projections of shoulder [(3), (4(ii))].

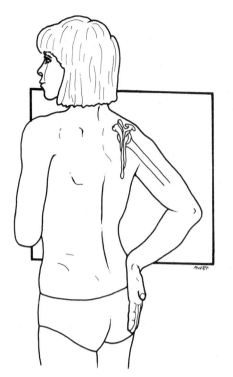

Figure 6.10. Position of the patient for projection (13)

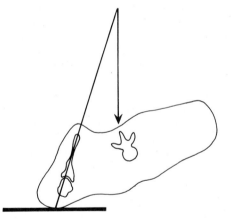

Figure 6.11. Position of cassette and production of profile projection of scapula from open X-ray tube diaphragms and midline centring point in projection (13)

(iii) Anteroposterior shoulder (projection (1)) with arm raised and hand resting on head.

Centre—Immediately below the outer third of the clavicle.

(17) Acromion process

This is demonstrated with the following projections:

(i) Anteroposterior shoulder (projection (1)).
(ii) Axillary projection of shoulder [projections (3), (4(ii))]. The process will be superimposed on the upper part of the humeral head.
(iii) Lateral scapula (projection (13)).
(iv) Lateral scapula for acromion. The patient is in the lateral position with the median sagittal plane parallel to the film. The injured side is nearest the film and the arm of the *affected* side is raised and folded over the head. Rotate the patient's trunk so the unaffected side moves forward through 20–30 degrees to show the scapula in profile.

Centre—To the medial border of the scapula at the level of the scapula spine.

Acromioclavicular joints

Both acromioclavicular joints should be examined for comparison.

(18) Anteroposterior acromioclavicular joints

Position as for anteroposterior shoulder (projection (1)).

Centre—Just above the head of humerus with a collimated beam. Repeat for other side.

Because of superficial position of the joint in the shoulder, the exposure should be reduced from that given to a routine anteroposterior shoulder projection otherwise the subject will be over-exposed. A grid is not necessary.

This projection usually results in the lateral end of clavicle being superimposed on the acromion. To avoid this use the same patient position but angle X-ray tube cephalad by 15–25 degrees. The degree of tube angle will vary from subject to subject.

(19) Alternative technique

This can be useful if the patient is round shouldered: the radiograph is taken with the patient in the posteroanterior position. A caudal X-ray tube angle may be required.

Subluxation

The patient should be erect for the anteroposterior view. Both joints are radiographed and then the examination is repeated with the patient holding a heavy weight, e.g. a sandbag in each hand. The joint space of the affected side may be seen to widen when placed under this additional stress.

Further proof of subluxation or dislocation may be gained from *tomography*.

Clavicle

The clavicle can be examined either in the anteroposterior or posteroanterior positions. Both techniques have advantages and disadvantages. Usually only one projection is required. A grid is not essential.

(20) Anteroposterior clavicle

Easier for injured patients although there is an increase in subject–film distance. The patient is erect or horizontal facing the X-ray tube, same positioning as for projection (1). (Alternative technique, projection (21).)
Centre—To the middle of the clavicle.

Children

Both sides can be taken for comparison.

(21) Posteroanterior clavicle

This produces a superior radiographic image to projection (20) because the clavicle is placed closer to the film.

The patient is erect facing the film. The head is turned away from the affected side. With a cassette placed in contact with the anterior aspect of the shoulder, better subject–film contact can be achieved than with positioning against a vertical bucky especially if the patient's arm is in a sling.
Centre—To the superior angle of the scapula. (The sternoclavicular joint is located at the level of the fourth thoracic vertebra.)

(22) Inferosuperior clavicle

This provides a second view of the bone, may be required to demonstrate displacement of fracture fragments or state of fracture union.

The patient is supine. The affected shoulder is raised slightly from the table on a non-opaque pad. The arm rests by the patient's side. The cassette is propped behind the affected shoulder and angled backwards 25 degrees from the vertical. The head is turned and the neck angled away from the affected side; the medial border of the cassette is placed well into the neck.

Centre—2.5 cm from the sternal end of the clavicle. The X-ray tube is angled 35 degrees from the horizontal towards the vertical (to be almost perpendicular to the cassette) and 15 degrees from the median plane towards the shoulder.

The second lateral angulation projects the sternoclavicular joint away from the vertebral column.

Sternoclavicular joints

Both joints should be examined for comparison. Because the joints are sometimes difficult to demonstrate with plain radiography, *tomography* is an important additional examination.

(23) Posteroanterior sternoclavicular joints

The patient stands facing the film, leaning slightly forward to bring the upper end of the sternum in contact with the cassette. Both shoulders are eased forwards slightly. Make sure the patient is not rotated, i.e. that the shoulders are equidistant from the film.

Centre—With a horizontal beam over the third thoracic vertebra. The focal–film distance is 150 cm. A grid is not required.

This projection does not demonstrate the joints clearly but it may give information about the symmetry of the medial ends of the clavicles. The radiographer may be aided by doing this projection before attempting the oblique views.

(24) Posteroanterior oblique sternoclavicular joints

The patient is erect or horizontal facing the bucky table.

For the right joint—The left side is raised from the bucky, rotated through 45 degrees.

For the left joint—The right side is raised away from the bucky, rotated through 45 degrees.

If the patient is horizontal the raised side must be adequately supported.

Centre—At the level of the fourth thoracic vertebra, over the raised side 10 cm from the mid-line with the X-ray beam perpendicular to the film.

Expose for each side in turn. The medial ends of both clavicles and the manubrium sterni are projected on to one side of the vertebral column on each film. The medial end of the clavicle of the *raised* side tends to be overshadowed by the sternum.

(25) Lateral sternoclavicular joints

The patient stands against the vertical bucky in the lateral position, i.e. the median sagittal plane of the body is parallel to the film. The affected side is nearest the film. The patient places his forearms behind his back and grasps each elbow. The shoulders are pulled well back.

Centre—With a horizontal beam over the sternoclavicular joints.

The subject–film distance is significant therefore a large focal–film distance is used (150 cm) to reduce magnification.

Sternum

Posterior to the sternum lies the mediastinum and vertebral column. The patient must be positioned so that although relatively close contact is maintained between sternum and X-ray table, there is minimal overlapping of the bone by these dense thoracic structures.

(26) Right posteroanterior oblique sternum

Patient erect or horizontal, facing the bucky table. Left side is raised, rotated through approximately 30 degrees. If patient is horizontal, raised side is supported on a non-opaque pad.

Centre—With the X-ray beam perpendicular to the film, 10 cm to the left of the fifth thoracic vertebra.

Diffusion technique

The sternum is a thin bone; when superimposed by lung tissue it has relatively low *subject contrast* and because of confusing lung markings it is difficult to see. A *diffusion* exposure technique can be used to improve the demonstration of the sternum. The aim is to deliberately induce movement blurring in the lung tissue whilst the sternum's position remains static. Immobilization of the wall of the thorax is vital; breathing will be mainly diaphragmatic. Horizontal positioning must be used and for added patient immobilization a broad bucky band is placed across the patient's chest. The patient breathes gently whilst a long exposure, e.g. 5 seconds, is used. The milliamperage is reduced accordingly.

Tomography

When using linear tomography, the long axis of the sternum should not be positioned parallel to the direction of the X-ray tube travel. Ensuring that it is not parallel reduces the effect of 'trailing shadows' produced by an overlying spine.

(27) Lateral sternum

The patient stands or sits in the lateral position, i.e. the median sagittal plane of the body is parallel to the film and the transverse axis of the sternum is perpendicular to the support. The shoulders are pulled well back.

Centre—With the X-ray beam perpendicular to the film, to the sternal angle.

The focal–film distance should be increased to 150 cm because of the large subject–film distance. (*See* projection (25).) Use a secondary radiation grid and expose the film on arrested inspiration.

Major sternal injuries

Where a patient has sustained serious thoracic injuries which may include a fractured and/or depressed sternum, the lateral projection has the greatest significance in diagnosis.

A radiographic examination of such a case could include:

(i) An anteroposterior chest radiograph.
(ii) A lateral sternum taken with a horizontal X-ray beam. Where possible the patient's arms are raised above his head to accommodate a shorter subject–film distance. A grid should be used.

This examination assumes that the patient cannot sit or stand because of his condition. In such a situation a posteroanterior oblique cannot be attempted unless special isocentric equipment can be used.

Ribs

The ribs are most frequently examined in cases of trauma and the *middle ribs* are more commonly fractured than the *upper* and *lower* two pairs. This is reflected by the relatively infrequent requests for examination of the latter.

Radiography of the thorax in trauma should not be undertaken solely to demonstrate the ribs. There may be abnormality of underlying structures, for example there may be a pneumothorax present. Positioning and exposure technique should therefore reflect awareness of this.

(28) Posteroanterior whole chest

The patient stands or sits facing the cassette. The chin is raised to rest on the top of the cassette. The upper border of the cassette must be high enough to include the first ribs and lung apices. The shoulders are pressed forwards against the cassette. The patient's elbows are flexed and the backs of the hands rest against the buttocks or alternatively the arms can be internally rotated and rest at the sides of the cassette. Check that the patient is not rotated.

Centre—With the X-ray beam perpendicular to the cassette, to the fourth thoracic vertebra.

On the film the scapulae should be shown clear of the lung fields. Exposure is made on arrested *full inspiration*.

A long focal–film distance (150–180 cm) reduces magnification of the posterior sections of the ribs.

Because of high inherent subject contrast, the desire for a short exposure time to reduce movement blurring and the large FFD, it is not usual to use a grid.

This projection will demonstrate the ribs above the diaphragm. The number of ribs shown may depend upon the degree of diaphragm excursion on inspiration. The high centring point tends to provide oblique rays which project the diaphragm downwards. Also demonstrated are the lung fields and the outline of the mediastinum.

Alternative techniques—projections (29(i)) and (29(ii)).

(29) Anteroposterior whole chest

(i) For a patient who can sit upright on a trolley but cannot support himself. The back of the trolley is raised and a covered cassette is placed behind the patient's back. His arms should be extended in front of him and internally rotated. He could hold the cot sides for support. The cassette should be high enough to include the first ribs and lung apices.

Centre—With the X-ray beam perpendicular to the film over the sternal angle.

150–180 cm focal–film distance. If the cassette is not vertical and the patient is not sitting upright then the X-ray beam must be angled downwards otherwise a *lordotic* projection of the chest will be produced, i.e. the ribs will appear to be horizontal on the film.

(ii) If the patient cannot sit up it may be possible to place a protected cassette behind his back if he can be gently lifted, otherwise a film may be placed in the bucky table tray and no patient movement is required. Exposure should be adjusted accordingly when using a grid. A larger subject–film distance is produced when using the bucky table therefore an extended focal–film distance is recommended (150 cm) to avoid projecting the thoracic wall off the film by the effect of magnification.

Pneumothorax

Where a pneumothorax is suspected but where it may be small, then a second film should be taken on *expiration*. Underpenetration of the chest walls is an exposure fault which may result in a small pneumothorax remaining undetected.

(30) Anteroposterior oblique ribs (projections (1–10))

In the anteroposterior or posteroanterior projection there is overlapping of the ribs in the axillary line. Fractures tend to occur in this region. This projection demonstrates the full length of the ribs on the side nearest the film. As the ribs slope downward a film of sufficient size should be used to include their upper and lower extremities. Adjacent ribs should also be shown as a fracture may also affect neighbouring bones.

The patient is erect or horizontal facing the X-ray tube. Rotate patient 45 degrees on to side of interest, raising the uninjured side. If horizontal the raised side must be supported. The patient's arms are raised and forearms should be folded over the head.

Centre—With the X-ray beam perpendicular to the film through the sternum at the level of the sternal angle.

A bucky grid can be used but is not always necessary. Expose on arrested *full inspiration*. The centring point is relatively high on the thoracic wall and produces oblique rays which tend to project the diaphragm downwards thus revealing more of the lower ribs.

(31) Anteroposterior oblique ribs (projections (9–12))

Because of the dome-like structure of the diaphragm the lower ribs are closely related to abdominal tissues. This situation is increased when the patient breathes out because of upward excursion of the diaphragm.

Although ribs 9 and 10 in part or whole can be demonstrated by projection (30) where they are overshadowed by less dense lung tissue, a second radiograph may have to be taken *adapting exposure technique* for abdominal conditions. The film will also show ribs 11 and 12.

Patient positioning is the same as for projection (30). Horizontal positioning may be preferred as abdominal contents tend to push the diaphragm to a higher level. Exposure is made on full *expiration* and a grid must be used.

Centre—Over mid-line at level of lower costal margin. With the X-ray beam perpendicular to the film. The low centring point produces oblique rays which tend to project the diaphragm upwards. Note that the film is not centred to the beam and that the lower border of the cassette is at the level of the lower costal margin. With X-ray beam collimators open to cover the subject and using an off-centred film, a large area of abdomen will be irradiated, and so this should be covered by lead rubber.

First and second ribs

In the posteroanterior chest radiograph (projection (28)) the upper two ribs tend to overlap. They are better demonstrated if the patient is horizontal.

The patient is positioned as for the clavicle (projections (20) and (21)) to demonstrate clearly the posterior and anterior extremities of the ribs, respectively. Where a stress fracture in the upper two ribs can mimic an apical lesion, *tomography* may be required.

Major thoracic injuries

Where damage to the lungs, pleurae or mediastinal structures has been sustained (this may have occurred *without* any bony injury) then the situation is potentially more life threatening to the patient when compared with the problems arising from simple rib fractures.

Assuming that the patient cannot be moved, the anteroposterior chest radiograph [projection (29(ii))] is likely to show rib fractures but should also demonstrate (if present) haemothorax, pneumothorax, any associated shifts in the mediastinum and also changes in the normal pattern of the lung markings.

The projection will not, however, demonstrate *fluid levels* although this may not be of prime importance at this stage. It is not usual or often possible to attempt oblique projections of the ribs in these cases; however, if this is required and the patient cannot be turned then an oblique view of the ribs can be taken by angulation of the X-ray beam across the patient. If a grid is used in this instance then it must be turned so that the grid lines run transversely in the direction of the tube angulation.

The bony thoracic walls are partly formed by the *sternum* and *spine*. In major thoracic injuries these will also probably require examination.

In some cases air infiltrates the tissues of the thoracic wall either because of the injury—*traumatic emphysema*—or after the insertion of a drain into the thoracic cavity during treatment—*surgical emphysema*. The amount of air present can vary but its presence has an effect on the radiopacity of the subject and exposures for the chest radiograph may have to be lowered.

Abdominal injuries involving lower rib fractures

Lower ribs can be demonstrated by projection (31). It may not be possible or desirable to rotate the patient towards his side, therefore a radiograph of the upper abdomen can be taken with the patient remaining supine. The lower border of the film corresponds to the lower costal margin. The cassette is placed transversely in the bucky tray so that the full width of the lower thorax is included on the film. Expose on full expiration, centring as for projection (31) and using lead rubber protection in the same way. If the patient is suspected of having abdominal injuries then the whole abdomen (and pelvis) will require examination.

Children and infants

A single anteroposterior or posteroanterior film is often all that is required for investigation of ribs in children. Although there is no exact age demarcation, older children may require oblique projections too.

Note that in children the thorax is short and wide when compared with the thorax of an adult. Movement blurring may also become significant, therefore choice of short exposure times becomes important.

Radioisotope scintigraphy

Rib fractures in some circumstances could be more easily detected on bone scintiscans than on radiographs[2].

References

1. COHN, R. (1972). Non-penetrating wounds of the lungs and bronchi. *Surg. Clin. N. Am.*, **52**, 585–95.
2. GRECH, P. (1981). *Casualty Radiology*, p. 214. London; Chapman and Hall.

7 The lower limb: foot to hip joint

Indications for the X-ray examination

The foot

The skeleton of the foot can be divided into two regions—the *forefoot* which consists of the navicular and cuboid bone and all the bones distal to them, and the *hindfoot* consisting of the calcaneus and talus. The forefoot inclines backwards and upwards, meeting the hindfoot at an angle and forming the *longitudinal* arch. This arch is high on the medial side but almost in contact with the ground on the lateral side. A second arch is formed by the metatarsal heads—the transverse arch. This arch is present only at rest and tends to disappear when the foot is weight-bearing. The bony arches of the foot are maintained by the actions of muscles, tendons and ligaments.

The tarsal bones each ossify from a single centre. Sometimes the posterior process of the talus is ossified from an independent centre and remains separated as an accessory ossicle, in this case known as an *os trigonum*. In all there are 29 different locations for accessory ossicles in the foot. As they are not always present bilaterally, radiographs of both feet may have to be taken to exclude a possible fracture.

Injuries

Fractures of the phalanges

These occur as the result of a crushing injury or 'stubbing' injury.

Fractures of the metatarsal shafts

These are usually due to direct violence such as from a heavy object falling on the foot.

March fractures

These are *stress* fractures that affect the neck of a metatarsal bone, usually the second or third. They occur where there is a flattening of the transverse mtatarsal arch so that the heads of these bones take an excessive amount of body weight (*see* also Chapter 2).

Fracture of the base of the fifth metatarsal

This injury is incurred when the foot is forcefully inverted. A piece of bone may be avulsed from the base of the metatarsal by the tendon of the peroneus brevis muscle which is inserted into it. This injury is often associated with a *sprained ankle*.

Fracture of the talus

Fractures vary in severity. Minor fractures such as a small chip or flake of bone (avulsion fractures) are most common. More seriously the neck of the talus may be fractured resulting in a disruption of the blood supply to the proximal fragment. This leads to *avascular necrosis* of this part of the bone with subsequent development of arthritis of the ankle and subtalar joints (*see* Chapter 3).

Fractures of the calcaneus

Caused by a fall from a height on to the feet. Minor fractures are usually just isolated cracks in the region of the tuberosity. In severe trauma the bone can be crushed and flattened—the degree of loss of the calcaneal angle gives an indication of the severity of the injury (*Figures 7.1 and 7.2*).

A fracture of the calcaneus may be accompanied by bony injuries elsewhere as the causative force is transmitted through the axial skeleton. The patient may also have a *crush fracture* of a vertebral body (upper lumbar is more likely) or a fracture of the base of the skull.

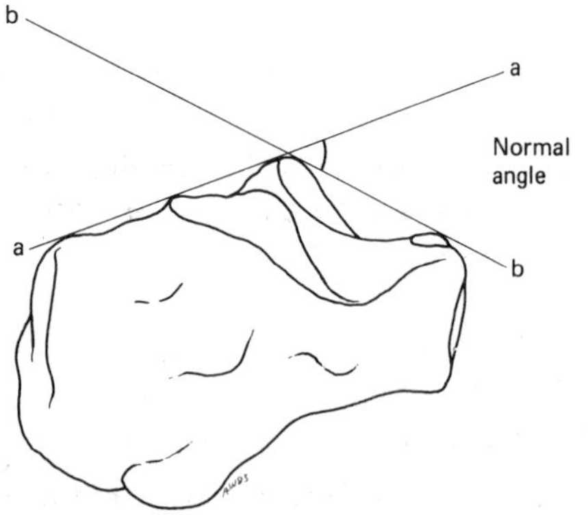

Other conditions

Hallux valgus

This is a common deformity of the foot, often hereditary. The big toe deviates outwards at the metatarsophalangeal joint and the prominent head of the first metatarsal bone becomes painful owing to rubbing of the shoe—a bursa or

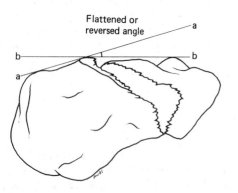

Figure 7.1. The lateral aspect of the right calcaneus showing the normal calcaneal angle

Figure 7.2. Fracture of the calcaneus causing reduction in the calcaneal angle

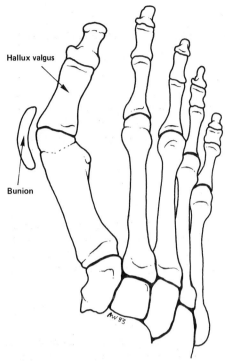

Figure 7.3. Hallux valgus

bunion is formed between the bony angle and the skin (*Figure 7.3*).

Treatment of this condition can be by *Keller's operation*—in which the prominent part of the first metatarsal head and the proximal third or half of the proximal phalanx are removed.

Metatarsalgia

This is pain under the metatarsal heads usually in overweight people. The pain is due to chronic strain of the ligaments supporting the arches of the foot.

Flat feet

Flat feet are caused by flattening of the longitudinal arch. This may be due to some structural abnormality of the foot—*pes planus*, or because, on weight bearing, the foot rolls inwards so that its medial border comes in contact with the ground. Since the hindfoot is everted (in valgus) this latter condition is known as *pes valgus*.

Raised longitudinal arch

This is the reverse of flat foot, the medial longitudinal arch is more concave than normal and the toes may be clawed. The term used for this condition is *pes cavus*.

Osteochondritis (see Chapter 3)

Osteochondritis affecting the foot includes:

(1) *Köhler's disease* affects the navicular. It usually occurs in children; the navicular becomes flattened and sclerosed so that it appears like a disc. Later, even without treatment, the bone reverts to its normal shape.
(2) *Freiberg's disease* affects a metatarsal epiphysis (the distal end), usually the second or third metatarsal.
(3) *Sever's disease* affects the apophysis of the calcaneum. An apophysis is a secondary centre of ossification taking no part in the formation of a joint—in this case of the posterior surface of the calcaneus.

Rheumatoid arthritis

Joints of the foot and ankle can be affected by rheumatoid arthritis, often early in the course of the disease. Gradual destruction of the joint surfaces leads to pain on weight bearing and the forefoot and toes can become severely deformed (*see* Chapter 3).

Sesamoiditis

This is inflammation of the sesamoid bone—often those behind the first metatarsophalangeal joint.

Congenital fusions

Fusion of certain tarsal bones can cause pain and deformity of the foot. Important fusions are:

(1) *Calcaneonavicular bar* seen in the oblique projections of the foot.
(2) *Talocalcaneal fusion* seen in the axial projection of the calcaneus.

See also Talipes, page 103.

Exostosis

A bony outgrowth relatively common in the big toe—usually from the terminal phalanx.

Spurs

A spur is a bony outgrowth which usually represents nothing more than a proliferative change due to stress from a tendon as in the case of an *Achilles spur* or at the attachment of the plantar aponeurosis of a *plantar (calcaneal) spur*. Spurs can be seen in profile on the lateral projection of the calcaneus.

The ankle region

The ankle or talocrural joint lies between the rounded upper surface of the body of the talus and the 'socket' formed by the distal end of the tibia and fibula. The joint is surrounded by a fibrous capsule supported by strong collateral ligaments.

The active movements at the ankle joint include dorsiflexion and plantar flexion. In dorsiflexion the angle between the front of the leg and the dorsum of the foot becomes diminished, in plantar flexion the angle is increased. It should be noted that inversion and eversion of the foot are brought about chiefly by movements at the intertarsal joints and not at the ankle joint.

Injuries

Sprained ankle

This is an injury sustained when the foot is forcefully inverted, the patient 'going over' on the outside of the foot. This may result in tearing of the lateral ligament of the ankle. The lateral ligament is in three parts:

(1) The anterior talofibular segment.
(2) The calcaneofibular portion directed downwards.
(3) The posterior talofibular segment directed posteriorly.

The first of these three parts of the lateral ligament is most likely to be torn and this injury is known as a sprained ankle. Often associated with this is a fracture of the fifth metatarsal base, although no bony injury is seen at the ankle. In more severe injuries the whole ligament may be torn.

Fractures of the ankle region

The range of combinations of ankle injury is large. Most involve fractures of the malleoli, with or without ligament damage. Some injuries are associated with a degree of subluxation or dislocation of the joint surfaces. There have been several attempts to classify these injuries and most of these classifications are based on the mechanism by which the injury has been caused. To simplify the subject, the

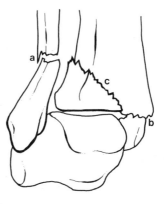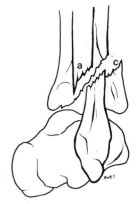

Figure 7.4. A trimalleolar Pott's fracture. The posterior and lateral aspects of the left ankle shows fractures through: **a**, the lateral malleolus; **b**, the medial malleolus; and **c**, the posterior malleolus

joint can be injured on either the lateral or medial side, or on both sides. In the most severe injuries both sides may be injured together with the posterior lip of the lower end of the tibia. This structure is often called the 'third malleolus' or posterior malleolus. There is a tendency to term most types of ankle fracture a *'Pott's fracture'* (*Figure 7.4*). The degree of severity is determined by the number of malleoli damaged. In some ankle injuries the interosseous ligament of the inferior tibiofibular joint is ruptured with separation of the two bones. This is known as a *diastasis*. The fibula may also be fractured at a higher level, e.g. the neck.

Other conditions

Talipes (club-foot)

A congenital deformity involving both ankle and foot. There are various types depending on the shape or position that the abnormal foot adopts.

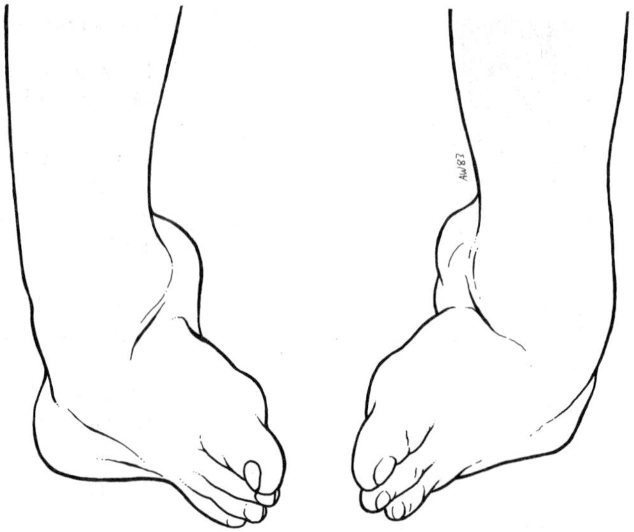

Figure 7.5. Talipes equinovarus

In *talipes equinovarus* (*Figure 7.5*) there are three major abnormalities:

(1) The forefoot is adducted.
(2) The foot is inverted.
(3) The foot is plantar flexed.

Treatment is by manipulation and splinting of the foot and ankle; and later, if necessary, by osteotomy.

The tibia and fibula

The proximal extremity of the tibia is expanded into two condyles and forms the knee joint with the femur. The tibia transmits the body weight to the ankle joint—a role in which the fibula plays little part.

Fractures of the shafts

These fractures are nearly always due either to sport or to traffic accidents. A large proportion of tibial shaft fractures are compound because about one-third of the bone is only covered by skin and subcutaneous tissue. Damage to the tibial arteries sometimes occurs and this may have to be assessed using *arteriography* in case resection of the arteries or amputation of the limb are necessary. The fractured tibia is often treated by open reduction and internal fixation. Sometimes there may be difficulty in union of these fractures because the tibial shaft has a poor blood supply particularly to its lower third. Treatment of *delayed union* is by bone grafting and internal fixation. Sometimes the healed fibula acts as a 'prop' keeping the tibial fragments apart so the surgeon may excise a short length of the fibular shaft to prevent this.

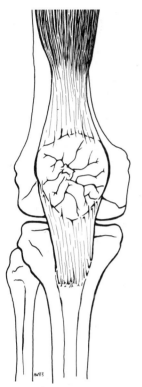

Figure 7.6. Stellate fracture of the patella

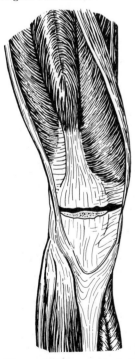

Figure 7.7. Transverse fracture of the patella with tearing of the patella retinaculum

The knee joint and patella

The knee joint is the largest joint in the body and is notable for its complex intra-articular structures. Lying between the articular condyles of the femur and tibia are the two radiolucent semilunar cartilages (menisci). The two cruciate ligaments lie in the central part of the joint and help to stabilize and strengthen it. The prime movements made by the knee joint are those of flexion and extension.

As the knee moves, a third bone—the sesamoid patella—glides up and down the patellar surface of the femur. The patella lies in the tendon of the quadriceps muscle and is linked to the tibia via the patella tendon. Occasionally a patella may ossify from two bony centres instead of the usual one and the centres fail to merge—*bipartite patella.*

A sesamoid bone may also be present in the outer head of the gastrocnemius muscle—the fabella—and is most easily seen on the lateral knee radiograph.

Injuries

Fracture of the lateral tibia plateau

A force that abducts the tibia on the femur while the foot is fixed on the ground may result in a fracture of the lateral tibia condyle. An example of this occurrence is when the bumper of a car strikes the outer side of the knee of a pedestrian. The lateral condyle of the tibia is compressed and depressed, usually becoming fragmented. This injury has been termed a *bumper fracture.*

Fracture of the femoral condyles

The fracture may involve one or both of the condyles. There is also a severe T-shaped fracture of the lower end of the femur which results in both femoral condyles being separated from each other and from the lower end of the shaft of the femur.

Fractures of the patella

There are two forms of fracture of the patella. The first is caused by a direct blow to the knee cap when the patella may break into several pieces. This is known as a *stellate* fracture but because the soft-tissue structures around the patella remain intact the fragments tend not to become separated (*Figure 7.6*).

The second form is the *transverse* fracture of the patella (*Figure 7.7*) and is caused by sudden violent contraction of the quadriceps muscle—as in attempting to preserve the balance after stumbling. The enormous muscle pull causes the bone to fracture transversely about its midpoint accompanied by tearing of the fibrous tissues (patella retinaculum) on either side of the bone. Wide separation of the two fragments usually occurs. In some individuals a similar force may result in rupture of the quadriceps or patella tendon instead of a fracture.

Dislocation of the patella

The patella can be dislocated from its groove on the femoral surface by trauma. Road accidents or sports injuries provide the usual cause and the patella is displaced either medially or laterally. In some patients, especially adolescent girls, *recurrent lateral dislocation* of the patella can occur. This is thought to be caused by certain inherent structural anomalies such as a shallow intercondylar groove and a small, highly placed patella.

Ligament injuries

A tear of the *medial collateral ligament* is caused by a stress that abducts the tibia on the femur. The joint is momentarily subluxed but when the patient is examined in the casualty department the subluxation has nearly always been reduced spontaneously. Whether or not the rupture is complete can sometimes be determined by taking anteroposterior radiographs while an abduction strain is deliberately applied to the tibia. If the tear is complete the knee joint space will widen at the medial side. Very wide abduction of the tibia on the femur cannot occur unless the *cruciate ligaments* and the *joint capsule* are torn as well.

A tear of the lateral ligament is much less common than that of the medial, and isolated tears of the cruciate ligaments are apparently quite rare. A sequel to a torn medial ligament is its calcification near the upper attachment; this is known as *Pellegrini–Steida's disease.*

Meniscus injuries

The menisci or semilunar cartilages are the remains of the complete cartilaginous discs which in fetal life separate the articular surfaces of the tibia and the femur. In the vertical section they are both triangular but they differ on the two sides in that the medial meniscus is *crescentic* in shape whilst the lateral meniscus is more circular.

Owing to the width of the pelvis, the femur normally makes a small angle with the tibia in the coronal plane. Most of the body weight passes through the lateral side of the joint and during rotation the lateral femoral condyle pivots on the outer side of the tibial plateau whilst the medial femoral condyle moves across the inner side. It is partly because of this relatively greater degree of movement that the medial meniscus is more likely to be injured than the lateral meniscus. This can occur when the knee is weight bearing, semi-flexed and the body is rotated. The semilunar cartilages are placed under a stress which could result in a tearing injury.

The menisci are radiolucent so they cannot be seen on 'plain' radiographs. A contrast agent (or agents) must therefore be introduced into the knee joint before they can be visualized in *arthrography*. A damaged meniscus may need excision—*meniscectomy*.

Other conditions

Osteoarthritis

The knee is the largest joint in the body and is subject to great mechanical stress therefore it is frequently affected by osteoarthritis. The degeneration is quite often secondary to some underlying cause—such as '*knock knees*' or '*bow legs*' where the arthritis develops in the half of the joint bearing the greatest weight. Sometimes operative treatment is carried out and this may involve *arthroplasty* (*see* Chapter 3). There are two types of knee prosthesis—one where the tibial condyles are replaced and another where new weight-bearing surfaces are given to both femoral and tibial condyles.

Loose bodies in the knee joint

For the description and causes of loose bodies refer to Chapter 3. Intercondylar notch projections of the knee joint may be required. Non-opaque loose bodies can be investigated by *arthrography*.

Rheumatoid arthritis

The knee is the commonest of the large joints to be affected by this disease. The patient complains of pain and stiffness in the joint and as the disease progresses the articular cartilage becomes damaged and this leads to a *secondary osteoarthritis* (*see* Chapter 3).

Osgood–Schlatter disease

The tibial tubercle is the commonest site for *osteochondritis* (*see* Chapter 3); both knees may be affected.

Genu varum (bow legs) and genu valgum (knock knees)

The distance between the hip joints is normally greater than that between the knees when the legs are together. Also, the femur usually makes an angle with the tibia in the coronal plane. Alterations in this angle are common and are usually termed knock knees or bow legs. These deformities can result from a disease producing weakening of the bones.

Examples are *rickets, osteomalacia* and *Paget's disease* (*see* Chapter 3). Changes in the joint ligaments have an effect on the bony relationships at the knee. Long continued stretching of the lateral side of the capsule accounts for the horseman's bow legs.

The femur and hip joint

The femur is the longest bone in the body, and because its shaft has a very thick cortex, it is also the strongest. The distal extremity of the femur is expanded into two condyles forming the knee joint with the tibia. The proximal end is characterized by the bony prominences—the trochanters. Directed medially and upwards from between the trochanters is the femoral neck with its rounded head. The head together with the bowl-like acetabulum of the innominate bone form the hip joint.

Injuries

Fractures of the femoral shaft

Because of the inherent strength of the bone, considerable force must be applied to it in order for it to break. A fracture of the femoral shaft tends to occur in road-traffic accidents and a patient with a fractured femur will probably have injuries elsewhere (some individuals may also have a *dislocated hip* on the affected side). The patient is likely to be severely shocked and in great pain, and despite the surrounding bulk of thigh muscles femoral fractures are often compound.

A fracture of the femoral shaft is most likely to be of the *transverse* type, and because there is no splinting action of a second parallel bone and because of the powerful muscles that span the bone, there is a characteristic angulation and overlapping of the two fragments. This displacement of the ends of the bone can produce a considerable degree of shortening of the leg, and the correction of this shortening is one of the main problems in the treatment of femoral fractures.

There are many different methods of treating this type of fracture. Generally speaking there are two approaches; the first involves placing the limb in some form of *traction* which has the effect of reducing the displacement of the fragments and then holds them in a position of re-alignment.

The average time for union to occur with this method of treatment is 6 weeks in a child and 12–16 weeks in an adult. After that, for about a month, a weight-relieving caliper may be used to protect the fracture when the patient walks.

An alternative method of treatment is by *internal fixation* using an intramedullary (Kuntscher) nail. This has the advantage of allowing rapid mobilization of the patient but carries the risk of infection. The nail is either introduced through the fracture site or through the upper end of the femur in a procedure carried out under X-ray control.

The methods used for treating adults may not be appropriate for children and infants. A device called the 'gallow's splint' may be used. In this technique adhesive strapping is applied to both lower limbs, and the child is nursed with both legs straight up in the air, the tapes being attached to an overhead boom; the child'sbody weight exerts a traction effect on the fractured bone.

Fractures of the upper third of the femoral shaft

These are comparatively uncommon unless the bone at this site is abnormal, for example where a secondary (metastatic) deposit from a carcinoma has caused a *pathological fracture*.

Supracondylar fractures of the femur (Figure 7.8)

Similar to fractures of the femoral shaft in that treatment is either by traction reduction or internal fixation. The lower fragment is displaced posteriorly because of the pulling force exerted by the gastrocnemius muscle.

The popliteal nerves or femoral blood vessels may be damaged at the fracture site.

Fractures of the neck and trochanteric region of the femur

Elderly patients tend to be most prone to fractures in the upper end of the femur. Although the term 'neck of femur' fracture is applied to most of these injuries there are in fact several distinct types of fractures grouped according to the level at which they occur. The exact site of the fracture has some bearing on how treatment will be carried out.

(1) *Subcapital fractures*—Where the neck of the femur joins the head. This type seems to be common in women over 60 years of age. There could be a combination of factors accounting for this—the bone may be weakened by *senile osteoporosis*, which tends to be more marked in post-menopausal women, also the angle between neck and shaft of femur is more acute in women, thereby throwing more severe strains on the femoral neck. Treatment of subcapital fractures is nearly always by internal fixation, e.g. Smith–Petersen nail. In order to obtain union of the fracture, perfect immobilization would be required and this is unlikely to be achieved by external splinting. Another important reason for not choosing extended immobilization of the patient is the risk to life from subsequent development of bed sores or pneumonia. The advantage of 'hip pinning' is that it allows the patient to become ambulant fairly soon after the injury, thus avoiding these complications and accelerating healing.

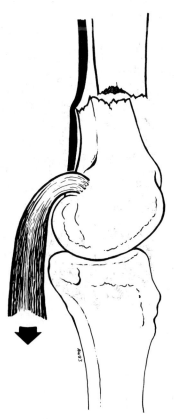

Figure 7.8. Supracondylar fracture of the femur. The gastrocnemius muscle causes displacement of the distal fragment

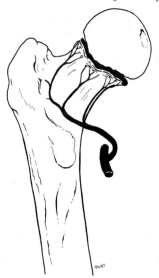

Figure 7.9. Disruption of the blood supply to the head of the femur as a result of a fracture through the neck

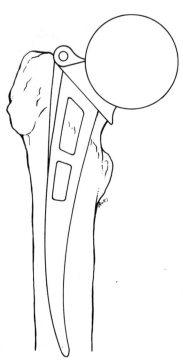

Figure 7.10. The Austin–Moore type femoral prosthesis

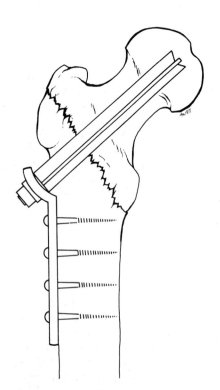

Figure 7.11. Nail and plate fixation for an intertrochanteric fracture

The blood supply to the head of the femur may be disrupted by the fracture (*Figure 7.9*) and there is a possibility of subsequent development of *avascular necrosis* in the femoral head (*see* Chapter 3 and also Hip Joint Dislocation, below). Even after the pinning the fracture will fail to unite; the head of the femur may collapse, often causing the nail to protrude into the acetabulum. To avoid this, instead of pinning the fracture the femoral head is excised and replaced by a prosthesis, e.g. Austin–Moore or Thompson prosthesis (*Figure 7.10*).

(2) *Intertrochanteric fractures*—Through the trochanters. At this site fractures occur with equal frequency both in elderly women and in elderly men. Intertrochanteric fractures are often *comminuted* and are usually fixed internally by a nail and plate (*Figure 7.11*). Although there is a good blood supply to this area of bone and the fracture would probably heal without internal fixation, the same dangers of immobilizing elderly patients for long periods remains.

In any variety of fracture of the neck of the femur, shortening of the limb is a rule. This is attributed to the tension of the powerful muscles with which the femur is surrounded. The untreated limb will also lie in *eversion*, and the patient will not be able to move the hip at all.

Hip joint dislocation

Comparisons are often made by anatomists between the hip and shoulder joints because they are both of the ball and socket variety. The shoulder joint, however, is much more frequently dislocated, because the glenoid cavity is much more shallow than the acetabulum.

There are two types of hip dislocation:

(1) *Posterior dislocation.* The head of the femur can be driven out of the acetabulum backwards if a force is applied along the axis of the bone when the hip is flexed and also slightly abducted. As this is the position a car driver adopts, a posterior hip dislocation is often the result of a traffic accident such as a head-on car collision.

(2) *Anterior dislocation.* The head of the femur will lie in front of the acetabulum. This type of dislocation is not so common.

To allow for the abnormal position of the femoral head both the joint capsule and the ligamentum teres must be torn. As these form the major route for blood vessels supplying the femoral head *avascular necrosis* may develop in this part of the bone (*see* Chapter 3). Radiographs are often taken of the hip at intervals for several months following such an injury so that any changes in the femoral head can be detected early, and *radioisotope scintigraphy* has also been used to confirm the presence of avascular necrosis. A dislocated hip can also be complicted by injury to the sciatic nerve which passes behind the femoral neck.

Fractures of the acetabulum

In about half the cases of *posterior dislocation* of the hip joint the head of the femur carries with it a fragment of bone from the posterior rim of the acetabulum. This is then known as a *fracture–dislocation.*

The roof of the acetabulum may be fractured if the head of the femur is driven inwards and upwards towards the pelvic cavity. There are several degrees of injury, ranging from a small crack in the acetabulum to a complete medial displacement of both acetabulum and femoral head—*stove-in hip.*

Other conditions

Osteoarthritis

The hip is the joint most commonly affected by osteoarthritis and whatever the cause may be, degree or severity of symptoms tend to influence the choice of treatment.

If a surgical method is chosen there are several techniques which include *arthrodesis, osteotomy* or *arthroplasty* (*see* also Chapter 3). Of these three major types of treatment interest has more recently focused on arthroplasty or *joint replacement.*

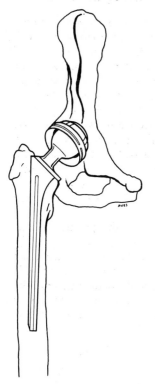

Figure 7.12. A total hip joint prosthesis

There are many different types of arthroplasty, usually named according to the surgeon who developed them. Some involve removal and replacement of the femoral head—Austin–Moore or Thompson prosthesis—although replacement of the femoral head alone is rarely successful in osteoarthritis since the acetabulum is also abnormal. Others involve removal and replacement of both femoral head and acetabulum. *Charnley* contributed much to this field and his arthroplasty consists of a femoral prosthesis articulating with a high-density polyethylene cup, both components being fixed in place using acrylic cement. There are several others types of arthroplasty based on the Charnley pattern (*Figure 7.12*). Charnley also pioneered the use of a separate operating enclosure to reduce the hazard of sepsis which apparently still remains the principal complication of the operation.

Rheumatoid arthritis

The hip joint can be involved—usually relatively late in the course of rheumatoid arthritis (*see* Chapter 3).

New growths

See Chapter 3, especially Osteosarcoma (page 37).

Tuberculosis of the hip

Tuberculosis of the hip usually commences from a bony focus, either in the femoral neck or acetabulum, from which it spreads to invade the joint cavity. The disease usually affects children who are often quite young. Early cases are treated by immobilizing the hip and by giving the patient appropriate antibiotics. If the disease remains untreated, destruction both of the bones and of the joint will result (*see* Chapter 3).

Congenital dislocation of the hip

This term is used to embrace a range of conditions where movement and stability of the hip joint are affected. True congenital dislocation of the hip, where the femoral head is displaced up out of the acetabulum at birth, is quite rare.

The cause of the condition is not known but diagnosis is very important because success in its treatment depends on early recognition. If treatment is not started and if instability persists the development of the acetabulum and the femoral head and neck will be affected. An early diagnosis from an anteroposterior pelvis radiograph is difficult because in the first few weeks the difference between the abnormal and normal appearances may be slight (the femoral head epiphysis will not yet have appeared)[1].

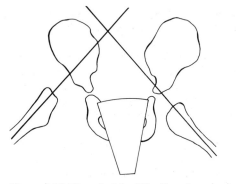

Figure 7.13. The principle of Von Rosen's projection

A special radiographic projection was proposed by *Andren* and *Von Rosen*. The baby is held in the supine position with both hips and knees fully extended; the legs are abducted each to 45 degrees and then fully internally rotated. The baby must lie symmetrically, immobilized by a bucky band, but should not be grasped too firmly above the hips because reduction of the affected hip may occur[1]. A line drawn up through the shaft of the undislocated femur (*Von Rosen's line; Figure 7.13*) if extended will cross the spine at the level of the lumbosacral junction. If the hip is dislocated the line will point outside the acetabulum and will cross the spine at a higher level. This technique appears to have fallen from favour owing to the problems of producing this projection accurately.

An alternative method of gauging the position of the femoral head is to refer to *Shenton's lines* (*Figure 7.14*). If the baby's legs are held together and the hips are extended when the anteroposterior radiograph is taken, it is possible on the radiograph to trace the line of the undersurface of the neck which when continued in the form or an arc is continuous with the undersurface of the superior pubic ramus.

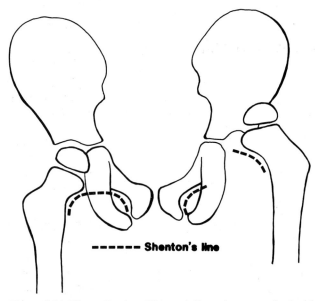

Figure 7.14. The application of Shenton's lines when comparing both hips

In the early stages, however, paediatricians rely mainly on clinical tests to determine the presence and degree of congenital dislocation of the hip rather than on radiographic examination. After about 4–6 months the femoral head epiphysis becomes visible and diagnosis from radiographs is more easily made.

Treatment initially consists of splinting the child's legs in abduction. There are many different types of splint; all of these hold the hip in the so-called 'frog' position. Traction may be used with older children but in all cases if conservative treatment fails then open reduction may become necessary. During treatment the radiologist will be asked to decide whether reduction of the hip has been attained or maintained. Where the patient is in a plaster spica, *tomography* may be undertaken so that assessment can be more easily made.

Sometimes it is the positioning of certain soft-tissue structures in the hip joint that prevents its reduction. *Arthrography* may therefore be required prior to operative treatment and can be used again in deciding whether complete reduction of a dislocation has been achieved.

Finally, the orthopaedic surgeon may reconstruct the acetabulum, thus making it more efficient. There are several operations designed to do this; one example is known as the 'shelf operation'.

Perthe's disease

This is *osteochondritis* of the epiphysis of the femoral head where the bone undergoes a characteristic cycle of changes which can be followed by taking serial radiographs of the affected hip(s). The cycle usually takes 2–3 years to complete. The epiphysis first becomes sclerosed, then fragmented and then subsequently returns slowly to normal. The shape of the epiphysis may become distorted and if this occurs the femoral head is usually permanently flattened (*see* Chapter 3).

There are a great variety of approaches to treating Perthe's disease, some being aimed at avoiding distortion of the femoral head and thus reducing the risk of later development of osteoarthritis.

Slipping of the upper femoral epiphysis (Figure 7.15)

This is a change in the relationship between the epiphysis of the femoral head and the metaphysis (or neck) of the femur. The epiphysis becomes displaced and comes to lie behind and slightly below its normal attachment to the neck. The displacement can be gradual or sudden and its degree is variable. The condition may not be apparent in the early stages on an anteroposterior radiograph, but may be best shown on the lateral film.

If gradual slipping is taking place and has been detected early, internal fixation with pins will prevent further displacement and stimulate epiphyseal fusion in an acceptable position. If the displacement is unacceptable, open reduction may be carried out followed by pin fixation. Slipping of the second hip may occur while the first is under treatment, so that both sides should be checked regularly. Some surgeons will also pin the radiologically normal hip to prevent it from slipping.

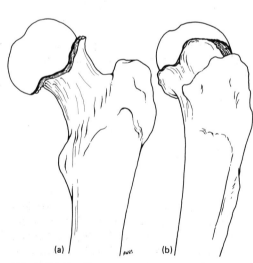

Figure 7.15. Slipped left upper femoral epiphysis. (**a**) Anterior aspect. (**b**) Lateral aspect

Coxa vara

This is not a disease but a *deformity*. The angle between the neck of the femur and the shaft is normally about 120–130 degrees; if it is *less than* 120 degrees the condition of coxa vara is said to be present. This alignment abnormality can be related to certain congenital conditions or can be the result of diseases where bone is softened, e.g. Paget's disease, osteomalacia. Mal-union of a fractured neck or trochanteric region of the femur is another cause.

Radiographic techniques

An exposure technique using a secondary radiation grid is generally unnecessary for radiography of the lower leg but owing to the greater volume of soft and bony tissue in the thigh, use of a grid is usually advisable for the femur and the hip depending on the subject size and type.

Foot

(1) Dorsi-plantar foot

The patient is seated on the table with his back adequately supported. Flex the knee and hip of the affected side and place the plantar aspect of the foot on the cassette. The opposite leg can act as a support.

Centre—With a vertical beam over the cuboid navicular region.

Both feet can be exposed on the same film where comparison is required.

Individual toes

Restrict beam size to include the affected toe and one (or both) of its neighbours. The metatarsophalangeal joint should be included.

Forefoot

The beam can simply be collimated to include only this area.

Hallux valgus

Examine both feet on the same film with the patient standing so the effects of weight bearing will be seen. Collimate the beam to include only the forefeet and centre between the heads of the first metatarsals. The X-ray tube is angled from the vertical about 15 degrees towards the patient's ankles.

(2) Dorsi-plantar oblique

There are two approaches to this:

(i) Position as for projection (1). The knee is then allowed to lean medially about 30 degrees from the vertical, the sole of the foot remaining flat on the cassette.
Centre: to the cuboid navicular region with the X-ray tube angled 15 degrees towards the ankle joint.
(ii) Position as for projection (1). The foot and leg are then tilted medially so that the sole of the foot makes an angle of 45 degrees with the film. Support the foot on non-opaque pads.
Centre: to the navicular with a vertical X-ray beam.

Both projections produce similar appearances—the tarsometatarsal articulations are more clearly seen than in projection (1).

Individual toes

Because the toes are not as mobile as the fingers they are difficult to demonstrate separately in a lateral projection. It is more convenient to use a dorsi-plantar oblique position to produce the second view of a toe or toes. This also allows for the proximal phalanx and metatarsophalangeal joint to be shown without being obscured by neighbouring bones.

Use the technique as for projection (2(ii)). Separate the toes if possible and if necessary with some non-opaque material. The sole of the foot must be adequately supported.

Centre—Over the first metatarsophalangeal joint for the great toe, and over the proximal interphalangeal joint for the other toes.

(3) Lateral foot

The patient lies on the affected side with the knee slightly flexed and supported. The lateral aspect of the foot lies on the cassette. The sole should be perpendicular to the film.

Centre—To the navicular cuneiform region with a vertical X-ray beam. This view gives further information in cases of tarsometatarsal dislocation and localization of foreign bodies.

Flat feet

A lateral of each foot is taken with the patient standing using a horizontal X-ray beam. A special cassette holder is used for this purpose.

Centre—To the lateral aspect of the foot. If the patient has to stand on the X-ray table make sure he is safely supported.

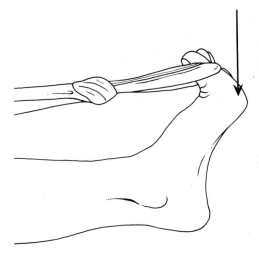

Figure 7.16. Position of the patient and direction of the central ray for demonstration of the sesamoid bones behind the big toe joint in the axial plane

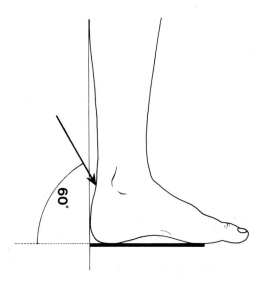

Figure 7.17. Position of the film and direction of the central ray in projection (5(ii))

Sesamoid bones

The sesamoid bones behind the first metatarsophalangeal joint can be seen on the lateral projection of the foot (projection (3)), and superimposed on the head of the first metatarsal bone in the dorsi-plantar projection (1). A third view can be obtained if the great toe is dorsiflexed at this joint and the X-ray beam directed tangentially to the posterior surface of the head of the first metatarsal (*Figure 7.16*). The sesamoids should be shown separated from the metatarsal.

Calcaneus

(4) Lateral calcaneus

Position as for projection (3). The sole of the foot should be perpendicular to the film.

    Centre—With a vertical beam, over the talocalcanean joint.

(5) Axial calcaneus

There are several ways of doing this second view of the bone but the following two seem to be the most useful:

(i) The patient is seated on the table with both limbs extended. The foot of the affected side should be dorsiflexed so the toes point straight upwards. To achieve this, place a bandage sling around the forefoot and ask the patient to pull gently, thus maintaining the position. The sling also helps immobilization. The lower border of the cassette should correspond to the lower border of the heel.
    Centre: to the plantar aspect of the heel with the X-ray tube angled 40 degrees cephalad.
(ii) The patient lies on the affected side. The unaffected limb is moved out of the way in front of the affected limb. Place a small pad under the lower leg of the affected side raising it slightly from the table. The cassette is supported vertically against the sole of the heel.
    Centre: to the back of the heel with a horizontal X-ray tube making an angle of 60 degrees with the film (*Figure 7.17*).

The foot should be at 90 degrees to the lower leg in either technique. This may not always be possible and sometimes a compensatory change in X-ray tube angulation can be made. In (5(i)) increase the angle towards the patient's head. In (5(ii)) increase the angle between the cassette and the X-ray tube. Both heels can be examined together for comparison on the same film using one exposure.

Talus and talocalcanean joints

The talus is demonstrated in the lateral projection of the hindfoot (projection (4)) where the beam size can be increased to include this bone. If an *os trigonum* is present in a case of injury a comparative radiograph should be taken of the other foot. The trochlear surface of the talus can be seen on the routine anteroposterior projection of the ankle (projection (10)). Although one aspect of the talocalcanean joints can be seen on projection (4), further projections are required to demonstrate them more fully.

There are three articular facets on the inferior surface of the talus with corresponding articular surfaces on the calcaneus. For the purpose of describing the techniques these can be considered to form the anterior, middle and posterior talocalcanean joints. (Strictly speaking the talocalcanean or *subtalar* joint is a single functional unit comprising articulations between the talus, calcaneus and the navicular.)

(6) Dorsi-plantar oblique

This demonstrates the *anterior joint*. Same position as in projection (2(ii)).

Centre—2.5 cm below and anterior to the lateral malleolus with a vertical beam.

(7) Medial oblique axial

This demonstrates the *middle joint* and also gives a tangential view of the convexity of the *posterior joint*. The patient sits on the table with the legs extended. The affected foot is dorsiflexed. If possible the foot is inverted. The leg is now rotated medially through 60 degrees and the foot is rested on a non-opaque pad.

Centre—2.5 cm below and anterior to the lateral malleolus with the X-ray tube angled 10 degrees cephalad.

This projection also shows the canalis or sinus tarsi 'end-on'.

(8) Anthonsen's projection

This demonstrates the *posterior* and *middle* facets. This can be used as an alternative to projection (7) and also shows the canalis tarsi. The foot is placed in the lateral position (projection (3)) with the lateral malleous next to the film. The foot is dorsiflexed.

Centre—To a point just below the medial malleolus. The X-ray tube is angled 25 degrees caudally and 30 degrees towards the toes. The focal–film distance is 35 cm.

These tilts may be impossible to produce together on many X-ray tubes. The foot position can be adjusted to counter this, but this now makes comparative reproduction difficult. The middle joint facet is also at its greatest distance from the film.

Projection (7) is considered to be superior to projection (8) because it is not only more easily reproducible but the sustentaculum tali (and hence the middle joint) is placed close to the film.

(9) Lateral oblique axial

A profile view of the *posterior joint*. The patient sits on the table with the legs extended. The affected foot is dorsiflexed. If possible the foot is everted. The leg is now rotated laterally through 60 degrees and rested on a non-opaque pad.

Centre: 2.5 cm below the medial malleolus with the X-ray tube angled 10 degrees cephalad.

Ankle

(10) Anteroposterior ankle

With the patient seated or lying the leg is extended with the toes pointing upwards. The back of the heel and ankle are placed on the cassette.

The foot ideally makes an angle of 90 degrees to the lower leg. To help achieve this a 45 degrees non-opaque pad and sandbag are placed against the sole of the foot. The foot is rotated medially until the malleoli are equidistant from the film.

Centre—With a vertical beam midway between the malleoli.

Because of the reciprocally curved surfaces of talus and tibia it will not be possible to demonstrate the talocrural joint space completely. It is more important to include the lower fibula and tibia on the film than the region below the malleoli.

The malleoli may be over-exposed where the subject is emaciated. A second anteroposterior view may have to be taken with a reduced exposure.

Patient in a walking plaster

This is a plaster-of-Paris splint which is constructed to allow the patient to walk. The plaster tends to be very thick and often a significantly larger exposure is required to penetrate it when compared with the 'average' plaster splint.

(11) Distal tibiofibular joint

Further information about the joint and the lower end of the fibula may be obtained by repeating projection (10) but with the leg rotated internally through 45 degrees.

Centre—Over the lateral malleolus with a vertical beam.

(12) Mediolateral ankle

The aim is to produce a projection which demonstrates the joint space between the trochlear surface of the talus and the inferior surface of the tibia. The medial malleolus will be superimposed on the lower end of the fibula.

The patient is rotated on to the affected side. Keep the affected leg straight at the knee. The unaffected leg lies behind the affected leg. The foot is dorsiflexed so that it is at 90 degrees to the lower leg. *Avoid* any inversion of the foot.

With the lateral aspect of the foot touching the cassette or table, medially rotate the leg slightly by about 15 degrees. This rotation superimposes the malleoli. The lateral aspect of the foot must now be supported on a pad.

Centre—With a vertical beam of the medial malleolus.

Alternative technique—projection (13).

(13) Lateromedial ankle

This technique is said to produce a better demonstration of the joint space.

The patient lies on the unaffected side. Bring the affected limb forward to lie on the table in front of the unaffected limb. The medial aspect of the foot and ankle lie on the film. Place a pad underneath the knee of the affected side for support.

Centre—With a vertical beam of the lateral malleolus.

Injuries

Modifications to technique may be necessary because the patient cannot move to facilitate the two basic views.

Two views must be taken at right angles to each other and the radiographer should at least attempt to produce an anteroposterior and lateral projection. If the patient cannot rotate the leg and body then the X-ray tube must be rotated around the axis of the leg accordingly.

With some patients it may sometimes be more convenient to take a conventional anteroposterior view and then turn the X-ray tube through 90 degrees for a lateromedial view. The cassette can be propped vertically against the medial aspect of the foot and ankle while the ankle is raised slightly on a non-opaque pad.

Ligament injuries

Damage to the lateral ligaments can produce instability of the talus within the ankle mortice (the 'socket' formed by the inferior surface of tibia and internal aspects of the malleoli).

A radiograph is taken of the ankle in the anteroposterior position (projection (10)). During the exposure the orthopaedic surgeon forcefully inverts the foot on the ankle joint. The talus will tilt outwards if the joint is unstable.

The procedure may have to be repeated with the other ankle for comparison. Lead rubber gloves and apron should be provided for the surgeon.

Tibia and fibula

The whole length of the two bones should be included on the film. More than one film (two separate exposures) may be required for each projection. In subsequent follow-up examinations it may be permissible to include only the joint nearest the lesion.

(14) Anteroposterior tibia and fibula

The patient is supine with the limb extended. The affected leg is rotated medially so that the malleoli are equidistant from the film. Immobilize the limb.

Centre—With a vertical X-ray beam midway between the ankle and knee joints.

The ankle and knee joints should be included on the film. If two films have to be used their positioning should overlap. After the initial examination, further radiological information may be gained by undertaking anteroposterior oblique projections of the lower leg. From the anteroposterior position the leg is rotated either medially or laterally by the required degree.

(15) Lateral tibia and fibula

From the anteroposterior position the patient is rotated on to the affected side. Flex the hip and knee slightly. The unaffected limb lies behind the affected limb. Make sure the patient has adequate support. The transverse axis of the patella should be 90 degrees to the film and the malleoli at the ankle superimposed.

Centre—With a vertical X-ray beam midway between the ankle and knee joints.

Injuries

Two projections must be taken at right angles to each other. Where a serious injury such as a compound tibial fracture has occurred, the limb tends to be externally rotated below the fracture.

Use a vertical beam for the first projection. Great care must be taken if a cassette has to be placed underneath the leg. It is preferable to use an accident trolley system which avoids moving the patient.

For the second projection, rotate the X-ray tube 90 degrees and direct the beam from the lateral aspect of the patient. The cassette is supported against the medial aspect of the leg. To include all of the knee joint and calcaneus it may be necessary to raise the limb slightly on non-opaque pads. Always seek advice and assistance if this is so.

(16) Proximal tibiofibular joint, head of fibula

This joint lies on the posterolateral aspect of the upper tibia. The limb must be rotated out from the anteroposterior or lateral position for the joint and head of fibula to be clearly demonstrated. There are two techniques:

(i) With the limb outstretched at the knee and the toes pointing upwards, medially rotate the leg through about 35 degrees.
Centre: with a vertical beam over the head of the fibula.
(ii) Position the patient as for projection (15). Now rotate the leg further laterally until the lateral border of the patella touches the cassette.
Centre: over the head of the fibula with a vertical X-ray beam. In this projection the head of the fibula is closer to the film.

Knee

(17) Anteroposterior single knee

The patient is seated or lying on the X-ray table with the leg outstretched and the toes pointing upwards. Medially rotate the leg slightly to centralize the patella over the lower femur. Immobilize the leg with sandbags.

Centre—2.5 cm below the lower border of the patella with the X-ray tube angled 5 degrees cephalad.

Make sure an adequate exposure is used. Underexposure of this projection is a common fault. If the patient cannot fully extend the knee use a curved cassette. Alternatively an ordinary 18 × 24 cm cassette can be placed with its long axis cross-wise, the cassette being supported on a pad behind the flexed knee. Although the length of bone shown is limited because the cassette is small, this method gives improved film–subject contact.

(18) Anteroposterior, both knees

With the patient seated or lying, both knees can be examined with a single exposure on one film. Placing a rigid piece of lead rubber vertically between the knees will prevent a lot of scattered radiation from reaching the film. This markedly improves radiographic contrast.

Prosthesis

Include the full length of the 'implant' on the film.

Weight-bearing anteroposterior knees

Where visualization of the alignment of the tibiae and femora is required a projection of the knees is taken with the patient standing.

A 30 × 40 cm cassette is placed transversely in a chest film holder or vertical bucky tray. The patient stands on a small step with both knees facing and touching the cassette or bucky. Patients for this examination are likely to be unsteady on their feet so it is wise to place them in a posteroanterior position where they can hold on to the support.

Centre—Between the knee joints with a horizontal X-ray tube.

If more of the limb bones are required on the film simply use a bigger cassette, e.g. 35 × 43 cm lengthwise.

(19) Lateral knee

From the anteroposterior position (projection (17)) the patient is turned on to the affected side. Flex the knee and hip slightly. The unaffected limb lies behind the affected limb. The transverse axis of the patella is 90 degrees to the cassette. The heel should be raised on a pad.

Centre—Over the medial condyle of the tibia with the X-ray tube angled 5 degrees cephalad. The tube angle compensates for the slightly lower position of the medial femoral condyle relative to the lateral condyle.

Weight-bearing lateral knees

Place a cassette in a film holder or vertical bucky. The patient stands with the lateral aspect of the knee next to the film. Flex the hip and knee of the unaffected leg and move it forward out of the way. The toes of the unaffected leg should rest on some immobile object but most of the body weight should be directed through the leg under examination.

Centre—With a horizontal X-ray tube over the medial tibial condyle.

Osgood–Schlatter's disease

Standard laterals of both knees are required for comparison, centring over the tibial tubercle and reducing the kVp by 5.

Injuries

The patient may be unable to turn on his side. Place a non-opaque pad under the knee and prop a cassette vertically against the medial aspect of the knee. Use a

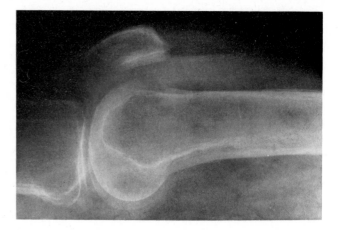

Figure 7.18. Lateral radiograph of the knee taken with a horizontal beam. A lipohaemarthrosis can be seen above the patella

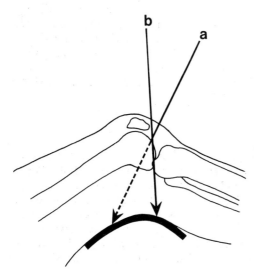

Figure 7.19. Position of the cassette and directions of the X-ray beam in projection (20(i))

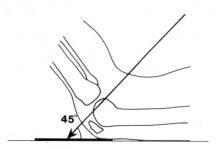

Figure 7.20. Position of the patient, direction of the central ray and position of the cassette in projection (20(ii))

horizontal X-ray tube and centre over the lateral tibial condyle.

A *lipohaemarthrosis* (*Figure 7.18*) indicates a fracture involving the joint. This can be seen on this projection because less dense fat floats on blood and forms a fluid level.

Arthritis

It may be more convenient for the patient if a lateral film with a horizontal X-ray tube is taken instead of using the conventional lateral position.

(20) Intercondylar notch

(i) The patient sits on the X-ray table with the leg in the anteroposterior position. Flex the knee over a curved cassette. Two films are taken.

Centre—Just below the lower border of the patella (*Figure 7.19*) with the X-ray tube directed:

(a) To make an angle of 90 degrees to the tibia. This shows the posterior part of the notch.
(b) To make an angle of 110 degrees to the tibia to show the anterior part of the notch.

(ii) This technique can be used as an alternative to projection (20(i)). The patient lies prone. Raise the lower leg off the table and flex the knee through 45 degrees and support. Place a cassette underneath the knee (*Figure 7.20*).

Centre—With the X-ray tube angled caudally 45 degrees, 2.5 cm below the crease of the knee.

The beam is directed along the axis of the notch. Both anterior and posterior margins of the notch are seen at once. Superimposition of the patella over the notch can be overcome by reducing the angle of knee flexion.

Patella

The patella is often examined in cases of trauma and care should be taken to avoid undue flexion of the knee as this may exacerbate an injury such as a *transverse fracture* of the bone.

(21) Posteroanterior patella

The patient lies prone. The leg is rotated so that the patella is centralized under the lower end of the femur. Place a pad underneath the ankle.

Centre—To the crease of the knee with a vertical X-ray beam. (Include the whole knee on the film.) This position is usually not possible in cases of injury.

Alternative technique—projection (22).

(22) Anteroposterior patella

Same position as in projection (17). Increase the FFD to 120 cm to compensate for the increased subject–film distance (normal distance between patella and film).

Centre—With a vertical X-ray beam over the patella (include the whole knee on the film).

The exposure should be increased from that required for a routine knee film.

(23) Lateral patella

From the anteroposterior position the patient turns to lie on the unaffected side. Position as for projection (19). This is more easily maintained if the knee is flexed slightly. The transverse axis of the patella is 90 degrees to the cassette.

Centre—With a vertical X-ray beam over the medial border of the patella. (Include the whole knee joint.)

With the knee straight the patella lies higher on the femoral patellar surface than when the joint is flexed.

Injuries

The lateral should be taken with a horizontal X-ray beam as in the case of knee injuries.

In patella *dislocations* it will be impossible to produce a true lateral of the bone. Where a patella is *bipartite* a radiograph should be taken of the other side for comparison.

(24) Inferosuperior (axial) patella

Also known as a 'skyline' projection. It is a supplementary technique where additional information is required about the bone and its sellar joint with the femur. The patient must be able to bend his knee.

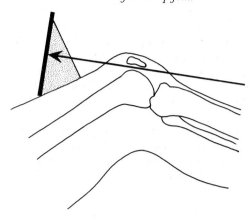

Figure 7.21. Position of the knee, direction of the central ray and position of the cassette in projection (24)

Sit the patient upright on the table and support his back if possible. Flex the knee to about 120 degrees. The patient holds the cassette, resting on a pad, at an angle behind the knee (*Figure 7.21*). The central ray of the X-ray beam is directed upwards along the vertical axis of the joint between the patella and femur.

Centre—To the apex of the patella.

It is difficult to specify the exact tube angulation as this depends on the degree of flexion at the knee.

Where axials of both patellae are required, a larger cassette is placed behind both knees which are exposed simultaneously, the centre lying between the knees. If the patient is not able to hold the cassette himself then a special film support should be used.

(25) Posteroanterior obliques of the patella

From the prone position (projection (21)) the leg is rotated 45 degrees first laterally and then medially. The knee should be flexed slightly. Support the foot on a pad.

Centre—With a vertical beam over the femoral condyle of the raised side in turn.

The medial or lateral side of the patella is projected clear of the femur. The exposure should be reduced by 10 kVp from the posteroanterior projection. Oblique projections are also used in *arthrography* examination of the knee joint. The degree of leg rotation is variable.

Femur, lower third

An anteroposterior and lateral with or without a horizontal X-ray beam are taken. The patient position is the same as for the knee simply using a larger film. Centre in any case over the condylar region of the femur.

Where the patient has an internally fixed supracondylar fracture include the whole of the 'implant' on the film.

Femur, middle third

Examined almost exclusively for fractures and their treatment.

(26) Anteroposterior femur

The patient lies supine with the hands resting on the chest. The leg is extended and the toes point upwards if possible.

Centre—With a vertical beam over the middle of the thigh.

Include both knee and hip joints on the film. Use two overlapping films if necessary, and use radiation protection on the gonads.

(27) Lateral femur

From the anteroposterior position the patient rotates to lie on the affected side. Raise the foot of the affected side on a small pad and flex the knee and hip. The sound limb lies behind the affected limb. The pelvis is tilted backwards 45 degrees so that the upper end of the femur is not obscured by soft tissues.

Centre—With a vertical beam over the middle of the thigh. Again include both joints on the film using more than one film if necessary. Carefully use radiation protection for the gonads where appropriate.

Injuries

Preferably, the patient should be examined with an accident trolley system. The anteroposterior film is exposed in the bucky tray thus avoiding moving the patient. A lateral of the lower two-thirds of the bone and knee joint is taken with a horizontal X-ray tube, the film being propped against the medial aspect of the leg. Even though a patient has a fractured femur the hip must *always* be examined. It is not possible to rotate the patient so a lateral projection of the upper third of the bone must be taken by other means (projections (32, 33)).

Patient on traction

Radiographs are taken to study the alignment of the fracture fragments and stage of healing.

For the anteroposterior view a cassette is positioned and supported under the affected leg. It may not be necessary to include both joints on the film. Centre the X-ray beam so that the central ray is perpendicular to the cassette. Take care to avoid pulling traction wires or displacing the traction frame when positioning the tube over the bed. A horizontal ray lateral of the middle and lower thirds of the femur is taken with the cassette positioned and supported against the medial aspect of the thigh. The lower corner of the cassette will have to be pushed downwards into the bed by the patient. Cover the cassettes in a pillow-slip.

If a metal splint is used (e.g. Thomas splint) then this may overshadow the bone but usually the alignment of fragments can still be assessed. If a lateral of the upper third of the femur is required this must be taken separately (projection (32)).

Femur, upper third and hip joint

Radiation protection is of importance in radiography of the hip region. Use of gonad shields, however, may be inadvisable at the initial examination.

(28) Anteroposterior single hip

The patient is supine with the legs extended. The arms are folded across the chest. The pelvis must not be rotated—the anterior superior iliac spines are equidistant from the film. The legs must be equidistant about the median plane of the body. The toes point upwards.

Centre—2.5 cm inferiorly along the bisector of an imaginary line drawn between the anterior superior iliac spine and upper border of the symphysis pubis of the affected side.

In young children it may be easier to locate the femoral pulse in the groin. The artery passes over the hip joint.

Acetabulum

For techniques, *see* Chapter 9.

Neck of femur and trochanters

The neck of femur is directed not only upwards and medially but also in a forward direction from the shaft of the bone.

This means that in the supine position where the toes are pointing upwards (projections (28, 29)) the neck of the femur is not parallel to the film. This produces a very slight degree of foreshortening of the neck of the femur.

If the whole leg is medially rotated this has the effect of raising the *greater trochanter* away from the film and reducing the foreshortening of the femoral neck. In injuries of the femoral neck or trochanteric region, the leg invariably falls outwards. This has the effect of increasing the degree of foreshortening but at the same time reveals the *lesser trochanter*.

Where comparisons of the two sides are made by referring to Shenton's line (*see* page 113), ideally both limbs and feet should be placed in the same degree of rotation although this is not always possible.

(29) Anteroposterior, both hips

Same position as for projection (28).

Centre—2.5 cm above the upper border of the symphysis pubis with a vertical X-ray beam.

Congenital dislocation of the hip

See page 112.

(30) Lateral single hip

From the supine position the patient is turned on to the affected side with the knee and hip flexed. The pelvis is tilted backwards through 45 degrees and supported. The sound limb lies behind the affected limb.

Centre—With a vertical beam to the upper third of the femur.

This projection of the hip and femur is not strictly at right angles to the anteroposterior view. This is achieved in projection (32).

Alternative techniques—projections (31–35).

(31) Lateral both hips ('frog's position')

The patient needs to have reasonable free movement at the hip and knee joints for this position. It is frequently used for children where comparisons of both sides are required. The patient is supine with the hands placed on the chest. The hips and knees are flexed. From position where the knees 'point' upwards the legs are externally rotated each through 60 degrees. The soles of the feet are placed together. The knees should be supported on pads.

Centre—With a vertical beam 2.5 cm above the upper border of the symphysis pubis.

If the neck of femur is of special interest the outward degree of rotation should be reduced to 15 degrees.

Injuries

The initial radiographic examination for fractures of the upper extremity of the femur should include an anteroposterior and lateral projection of the hip. The lateral film is vital in the case of an *impacted fracture* of the neck of femur because it may not be apparent from the anteroposterior film. It is also usual to take an anteroposterior view of the whole pelvis because the patient may have sustained other bony injuries such as a fracture of the pubic rami. As so many of these patients are elderly and are most likely to have operative treatment, a routine chest radiograph taken at the same time avoids another trip to the department for the patient.

(32) In cases of injury where the patient cannot be rotated, or when following up operative treatment

The patient remains supine. A cassette and grid is propped vertically against the affected side of the patient. The uppermost edge is pressed well into the patient's waist. The long axis of the cassette is parallel to the neck of the femur.

Raise the sound limb from the table, flexing the knee and hip. The sound limb is rotated outwards at the hip joint and the foot should come to rest on the light-beam collimator box of the X-ray tube.

Direct a horizontal X-ray beam from the unaffected side of the patient to be perpendicular to the neck of the femur. Collimate the beam as much as possible (*Figure 7.22*).

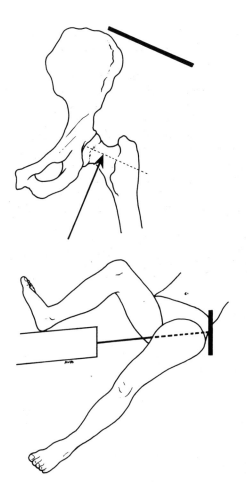

Figure 7.22. Positions of patient, film and direction of the X-ray beam in projection (32)

Adequate flexion and external rotation of the sound hip is important in order to avoid superimposition of soft-tissue shadows of this leg over the head of femur on the side of interest.

(33) Where the sound leg cannot be raised and the patient must not be rotated

The cassette and grid is placed in the same position as for projection (32) except that the cassette is tilted backwards by 25 degrees and supported (*Figure 7.23*). The X-ray tube is directed towards the neck of the femur as in projection (32) except an additional tilt of 25 degrees (vertically towards the floor) is made.

The cental ray should be perpendicular to the cassette. This is of special importance where a grid is used.

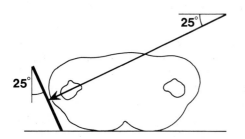

Figure 7.23. Position of cassette in projection (33)

(34) If the sound leg cannot be raised but the trunk can be turned slightly

From the anteroposterior position the pelvis is tilted so the hip under examination is raised above the level of the sound hip. Support the raised side on non-opaque pads. The cassette and grid are propped vertically against the outer aspect of the hip, its top edge pressed into the patient's waist. The long axis of the film is parallel to the femoral neck.

Centre—With a horizontal X-ray beam towards the upper end of the femur so the central ray is perpendicular to the cassette (*Figure 7.24*).

An example of a use for this technique is where the hips are immobilized in a plaster spica.

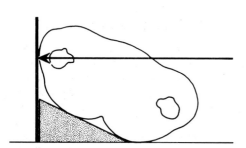

Figure 7.24. Position of cassette in projection (34)

(35) Another method of producing a lateral view of the hip

The patient sits with his knees flexed over the end of the table. The cassette and grid is vertically supported at the side of the thigh and hip (*Figure 7.25*).

Centre—With a horizontal X-ray beam from between the legs towards the neck of femur.

This could be the projection of choice where the patient cannot easily lie down or where there is limited movement at the hips.

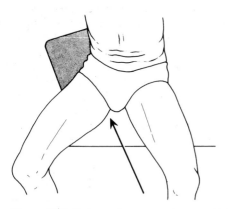

Figure 7.25. Position of cassette and centre of beam in projection (35)

Theatre procedure for hip pinning

'Hip pinning' refers to open reduction and internal fixation of fractures of the femoral neck or trochanteric region. Either conventional radiography or fluoroscopy with image intensification is used to produce a series of anteroposterior and lateral projections of the neck of the femur during the operation.

Essentially, the surgeon needs to monitor the direction and the placing of the nail. If a femoral plate is used then the angle it will make with the nail has to be carefully measured. Anteroposterior and lateral radiography or fluoroscopy of the affected hip will be undertaken at the following stages of the operation:

(1) Before the operation starts when the anaesthetized patient is on the theatre table. This is in order to check the current position and state of the fracture fragments.
(2) After the insertion of the guide wires to determine the best route for the insertion of the implant.
(3) After the positioning and fixation of the implant.

The advantage of using films rather than fluoroscopy is that they act as a permanent record of the operation; and even if image intensification has been used, final radiographs ought to be taken before the patient leaves the theatre for the ward.

Limb length discrepancy and its assessment

Poliomyelitis is a rare viral infection where the anterior horn cells of the spinal cord are selectively attacked resulting in muscular paralysis. If the resultant weakness of the lower limb muscles is extensive it may result in retardation of growth, the child ending the growth period with the affected limb shorter than the normal one. Polio is one cause of leg shortening encountered in orthopaedics. Other causes are fractures, chronic hip disease, congenital shortening and damage to the epiphyseal plate.

There are two ways of dealing with leg length discrepancy: either to shorten the longer limb or lengthen the shorter one. Most surgeons prefer to lengthen the shorter limb as this avoids operating on a normal leg.

Either the femur or tibia is lengthened. The bone is osteotomized then gradually distracted by up to 5 cm. New bone is laid down between the cut ends. In the case of the tibia, the fibula has also to be osteotomized at the same time. Limb length discrepancy can also be treated by temporarily stopping growth at the lower femoral and upper tibial epiphyseal plates. This is achieved by placing staples across the growth plate, one prong being in the epiphysis and the other in the metaphysis. The staple can be removed at any time and growth then recommences provided no damage has been done to the growth plate.

Accurate radiographic measurement of limb length is required before and during corrective treatment. The surgeon needs to know the exact length of the limb components. In a standard radiograph of a long bone the divergent X-ray beam produces elongation where the centring point is the middle of the shaft. Special equipment and techniques have been devised to side-step this problem.

One method is to use a rectangular plastic grid. Inside and across the narrower dimension are set lengths of metal wire spaced at centimetre intervals. Lead numbers are placed along one long side marking the grid into 10 cm lengths. The grid is placed on the surface of the X-ray table, parallel to and central around the long axis of the table. The patient lies supine with both legs extended on the grid. The hip joints should be below the grid's upper level and the pelvis must be in the true anteroposterior position (*see* Projection (1), page 164). The legs should be centralized on the grid and the toes should point upwards.

Six separate exposures are made centring *accurately* over the right and left hip joint, knee joint and ankle joint in turn. A 35 × 43 cm cassette is placed in the bucky tray. For the hip joint exposures the upper border of the film corresponds to the upper end of the plastic grid. For the knees the cassette is moved so that its centre is at the level of the joints. Finally, for the ankle the casstte's lower border lies at the level of the lower edge of the measuring grid.

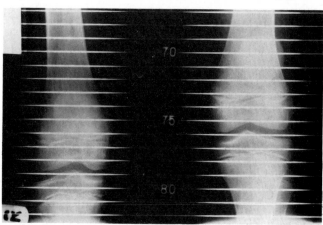

Figure 7.26. Radiograph of both knees taken during limb length measurements. In this instance both joints have been recorded using a single exposure. The grid lines are spaced at 1 cm intervals and numbered at 5 cm intervals

The patient must be adequately immobilized and must be encouraged or assisted not to move between exposures. The spaced wires are superimposed on the joints and some of the lead numbers will have been exposed by the radiation fields. Measurement readings of leg length can now be taken (*Figure 7.26*).

A preferable method for young children who may be difficult to immobilize is to take a single radiograph using a large focal–film distance—*teleradiography*. This will require a special cassette, e.g. 100 cm long. A single exposure is made with the beam centred at the mid-point of the lower limbs. This method has the advantage of showing the full length of the limbs and the alignment of the bones.

Reference

1. SUTTON, D. (1980). *A Textbook of Radiology and Imaging*, 3rd edn, pp. 4–6. Edinburgh; Churchill Livingstone.

8 The vertebral column

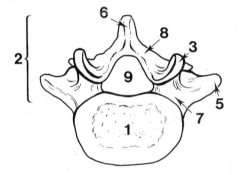

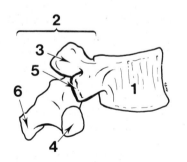

Figure 8.1. Superior and lateral aspects of a typical lumbar vertebra: 1, body; 2, neural arch; 3, superior articular process; 4, inferior articular process; 5, transverse process; 6, spinous process; 7, pedicle; 8, lamina; and 9, vertebral foramen

The vertebral column is a complex anatomical structure. Part of the axial skeleton, it plays a role in transmission of body weight via the sacroiliac joints to the pelvis and lower limbs.

The vertebral column is divided into five regions: the uppermost and more mobile cervical spine, the dorsal spine with which the ribs are articulated, the more massive lumbar spine, the fused sacral vertebrae and the rudimentary 'tail' (the coccyx). There are 33 vertebrae in all—seven cervical, twelve dorsal, five lumbar, five sacral and four coccygeal. Individual vertebrae can be conveniently referred to by naming each bone with a letter and number, e.g. the second lumbar vertebra can be termed L2.

Except for the uppermost two vertebral bones, the cervical, dorsal and lumbar vertebrae are all roughly the same shape (*Figure 8.1*). A cylindrical body lies at the front forming symphyseal-type (anterior) joints with the bodies of the adjacent vertebrae. Posteriorly is the neural arch which encloses the spinal cord or nerves and meninges. Each neural arch has a pair of superior and inferior articular processes which form synovial plane (posterior) joints with the processes of the bones above and beneath it.

Indications for the X-ray examination

The cervical spine

Cervical spine injuries

Injuries to the cervical spine are common and tend to occur in falls and in road-traffic accidents. Neck injuries are often found in combination with head injuries and are therefore sometimes difficult to assess by the medical staff because the patient may be unconscious at the time of examination. These patients must be handled with care during the initial X-ray examination and until the extent of damage is known.

In all injuries to the vertebral column there is always a danger of damage to the spinal cord. This damage may be in the form of interference with the blood supply, compression, contusion (bruising) or transection (tearing). In the cervical spine the canal is fairly wide so there is a greater chance of the cord escaping severe damage than if the injury were in a lower part of the spine. If cord injury does occur the outcome will either be fatal or the patient may have some degree of quadriplegia. The phrenic nerve provides the motor supply to the diaphragm and arises mainly from the fourth cervical segment (at about the level of the body of C4). Any injury to the spinal cord above this level may cause immediate cessation of respiration and death.

The upper limbs are innervated by the fifth cervical to the first thoracic segments via the brachial plexus. If the patient has injury at a lower cervical level (a common site) then the patient may have quadriplegia but it is still possible for a good deal of arm function to remain.

Injuries of the cervical spine are grouped according to the mechanism that caused them. Traumatologists refer to *flexion* and *extension injuries*—although rotational forces may also play a part. The *whiplash injury* is common in motorists whose cars are 'shunted' from behind while stationary. The mechanism of this injury includes both flexion and extension components.

Because the posterior intervertebral joints are more horizontally inclined and laterally placed in comparison with the same joints in the rest of the spine, subluxations and dislocations of these facet joints are far more common than elsewhere. Forceful flexion of the neck may cause subluxation of one or both of a pair of joints. This is not serious but it may cause irritation of a nerve root leading to pain in the arm or side of the neck. The lateral radiograph may show malalignment of the vertebrae. A more serious flexion injury involves true dislocation of the posterior intervertebral joints (*Figure 8.2*) with or without a crush fracture of a vertebral body.

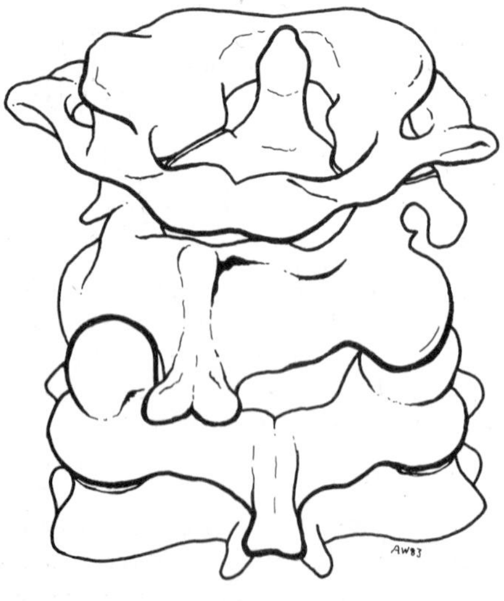

It should be emphasized that the degree of anatomical abnormality demonstrated on the X-ray films may not bear any relationship to the degree of cord damage present. Dislocation of the posterior vertebral joints may result in quadriplegia for the patient but the radiograph may be 'normal' because the dislocation has undergone a spontaneous reduction.

Treatment of dislocation of the intervertebral joints can be carried out by traction using skull calipers inserted under general anaesthetic followed by immobilization.

Figure 8.2. Posterior aspect of the upper cervical vertebrae, showing dislocation of an intervertebral joint on one side

Extension injuries may cause tearing of the spinal longitudinal ligaments. Fracture of the lower spinous processes and neural arches may sometimes occur in whiplash injuries when the head is driven backwards.

Fracture of the atlas (Jefferson fracture)

This is a rare injury where a vertical blow to the head splits the atlas so both lateral masses are displaced sideways (*Figure 8.3*). This is often caused by impact of the head on the bottom of a swimming bath after a dive and in some cases will cause immediate death because of cord compression.

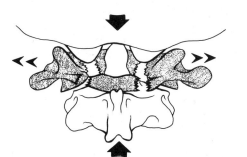

Figure 8.3. Jefferson fracture of the atlas. Forces directed along the axial skeleton results in the 'splitting' of the bone

Posterior arch of the atlas fracture

Owing to hyperextension of the neck, the arch is compressed between the occiput and the posterior arch of the axis.

Fracture of the axis (Figure 8.4)

Fractures usually occur at the base of the odontoid peg with displacement of the fragment together with the atlas in either a forward or backward direction. This is an injury

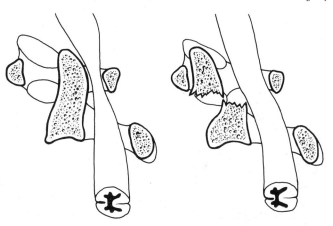

Figure 8.4. (*Left*) Rupture of the transverse ligament causing dislocation of the entire axis. (*Right*) Fracture at the base of the odontoid peg with posterior displacement of the rest of the bone

from which the patient usually survives. If there is a rupture of the transverse ligament of the atlas, which crosses immediately behind the peg, then the atlas can be dislocated and the outcome may be fatal cord compression.

Cervical spine dislocations in children

Spontaneous dislocation—especially of the atlas—can occur in children who have recently had a throat infection. The dislocation is due to changes in the soft-tissue structures of the spine and is treated by traction and immobilization.

Other conditions

Cervical spondylosis

Spondylosis is a term used particularly to describe degeneration of the intervertebral discs although there is often osteoarthrosis also present in the joints between the articular facets. Cervical spondylosis is probably the commonest cause of the syndrome of neck and upper arm pain. It tends to affect the vertebral joints between the fifth, sixth and seventh cervical vertebrae. (*See* also Lumbar spondylosis, page 141.)

Radiographs may show some narrowing of the disc spaces and in later cases the presence of osteophytes attached to the vertebral bodies. Osteophytic encroachment produces narrowing of the intervertebral foramina which may lead to pressure on the nerve roots and thus to symptoms of pain (neuralgia) in the area of the nerve's distribution.

Cervical disc prolapse

Wear and tear seems to have more effect on the lower region of the cervical vertebra, and the intervertebral discs that are involved in spondylosis are also the ones most likely to prolapse.

This condition is not as common in the cervical spine as it is in the lumbar region but the disc lesion is the same in either case (*see* page 141). Irritation of a nerve root caused by the prolapsed disc may result in the patient experiencing pains radiating down the arm (*brachial neuralgia*). This pain may be severe and some surgeons advise removal of the disc material and bone grafting of the disc space.

Torticollis

This is a condition in which the neck lies in abnormal lateral flexion with both the head and the neck also rotated to the same side.

Torticollis may be caused by spasm in the sternomastoid and trapezius muscles following trauma to the neck. It is also often associated with cervical disc prolapse. *Congenital torticollis* is not a true developmental defect, but it is due to a birth injury that causes fibrosis in one sternomastoid muscle and as a result during growth a torticollis forms. If this is left untreated the face and the jaw will become asymmetrical.

Thoracic outlet syndrome

Compression of the subclavian artery and the lower trunk of the brachial plexus may cause symptoms to arise in the limb of their supply. The area bounded by the first ribs is known as the thoracic outlet and symptoms arising from causes in this area are referred to as the thoracic outlet syndrome. The vessel and nerve trunk may be compressed by the tightness of the scalene muscles or by the presence of a supplementary rib arising from the seventh cervical vertebra. *Cervical ribs* vary greatly in size and shape and clinical symptoms bear little relationship to the radiographic abnormality. A very small cervical rib may have a fibrous band attachment which causes much disability for the patient, whereas a large rib may produce no problems at all. Narrowing of the subclavian artery may be demonstrated by angiography.

Rheumatoid arthritis

This can cause instability of the atlantoaxial joints. Symptoms of pressure on the spinal cord may provide the first evidence of the disease (*see* Chapter 3).

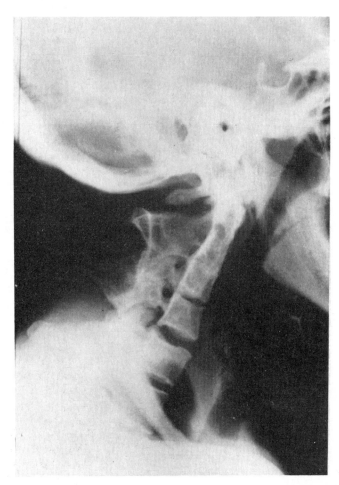

Figure 8.5. Lateral radiograph of the cervical spine in Klippel–Feil syndrome

New growths

See page 144.

Separate odontoid process (os odontoideum)

This is a congenital condition where the odontoid peg is completely detached from the body of the second cervical vertebra and lies situated in the region of the foramen magnum.

Klippel–Feil syndrome (Figure 8.5)

This is a developmental defect where many cervical vertebrae are fused, the neck is short and its movements are restricted. Other congenital anomalies such as *Sprengel's shoulder* (*see* Chapter 6), *spina bifida* and rib lesions usually coexist.

The thoracic spine

Injuries

See page 144.

Other conditions

Kyphosis

The normal backwards curve of the thoracic vertebrae is called the thoracic *kyphosis*; however, the term can also be used to denote an abnormally accentuated curve.

There are several pathological causes of this deformity. If a vertebral body collapses and becomes wedge shaped as a result of trauma or pathology then there tends to be an associated angular increase in the curve. This is known as a *kyphos* or *gibbus*. If pathological involvement includes several or all of the vertebral bodies then there will be a general rather than an angular increase in the curvature, e.g. in *ankylosing spondylitis*, *Paget's disease* and *osteoporosis* (*see* Chapter 3).

Senile kyphosis

In old age some individuals tend to develop a kyphosis and consequently lose height. This can be because of a combination of vertebral flattening and wedging as the bones undergo changes of *senile osteoporosis* (*see* Chapter 3).

Intervertebral discs also have a tendency to become reduced in thickness as age advances and this partially accounts for the loss in height.

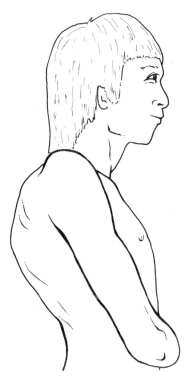

Figure 8.6. Adolescent kyphosis

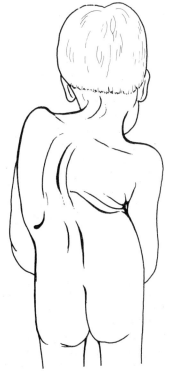

Figure 8.7. Idiopathic scoliosis

Adolescent kyphosis (Figure 8.6)

In the 1900s Scheuermann described a condition that causes an increase in the normal anteroposterior curve of the thoracic spine in adolescents.

Until puberty the upper and lower surfaces of the vertebral bodies are cartilaginous. At this time two annular epiphyses for the circumferential parts of the upper and lower surfaces of the body appear. These secondary centres fuse with the rest of the bone at about the age of 25 years. In adolescent kyphosis these annular epiphyses seem to develop abnormally so the vertebral bodies fail to grow properly and become wedge shaped. This view is apparently controversial and other authorities think that the changes are due to herniation of the nucleus of the intervertebral disc into the adjacent vertebral bodies—*Schmorl's nodes*—and narrowing of the disc spaces.

Scoliosis

Scoliosis is a complex condition which is most simply defined as a lateral curve or tilt of a part of the spine. In addition to this lateral curvature there is often also a rotation of the vertebral column around its longitudinal axis. If the scoliosis is in the thoracic spine the ribs are distorted by the rotation, producing a hump on one side. This deformity of the chest cage may interfere with lung function. Patients with severely deformed chests are more prone to recurrent chest infections. These and other structural changes and defects are part of what is known as *structural scoliosis*. In most of these cases there is no known cause—*idiopathic scoliosis (Figure 8.7)*. Other structurally scoliotic spines can be attributed to some congenital defect or neuromuscular problem.

The basis of treatment is to attempt to hold the curve by external splintage as long as possible, then to fuse the spine surgically when the child is old enough to have achieved reasonable growth. There are many types of external splint; the most successful is the *Milwaukee brace* which exerts pressure on the iliac crests with a counter-pressure under the occiput and chin.

Non-structural scoliosis is when the curve is flexible and corrects when the patient bends to the convex side. The commonest cause of this condition is the natural attempt to compensate for an irregularity in leg length. Spasm of the spinal muscles associated with a prolapsed intervertebral disc is another cause of non-structural scoliosis.

Tuberculosis of the spine (Pott's disease)

The spine is the commonest part of the skeletal system to be affected by tuberculosis. The original focus of the disease is in a vertebral body from where it spreads and destroys the neighbouring disc and adjacent vertebral body. As the bone collapses it may produce an angular deformity of the spine (kyphos). A paravertebral abscess is formed which surrounds the vertebral bodies. In the lower dorsal and lumbar regions, pus may spread into the neighbouring psoas muscle sheath to form a psoas abscess. If the disease in the thoracic region spreads posteriorly, the spinal canal may become narrowed and pressure on the spinal cord may result in *Pott's paraplegia*.

New growths

See page 144.

The lumbar spine

Injuries

See page 144.

Other conditions

Lumbago and sciatica

Lumbago means low back pain. This is a very common complaint which has a variety of causes, some not necessarily located in the spine. In a large number of instances there is a specific cause, but often no abnormality is found. Individuals with 'mechanically weak' spines appear to have a greater tendency to suffer from backache. Mechanical weakness may be brought about by some minor structural anomaly (quite common in the lumbosacral region) or some degree of muscular inefficiency. An acute attack of lumbago—pain and muscle spasm—may be experienced in *lumbar disc prolapse*.

For patients with chronic back pain radiographic examinations may help to find the cause of the problem. Films may show the minor structural changes already mentioned but may also demonstrate degenerative changes (spondylosis) or other bony pathology. Secondary neoplastic disease may have to be investigated by taking radiographs of other parts of the body. Lesions involving non-radiopaque structures such as spinal nerves and intervertebral discs may require contrast studies.

Renal pathology may cause back pain; however, this and other extra-spinal causes of back pain are usually excluded by clinical means as well as by radiology.

Sciatica or *sciatic neuralgia* is characterized by pain radiating to the leg. The chief cause is compression of one of the lumbar nerve roots. This can occur in *lumbar disc prolapse* or because of osteophytic encroachment of the intervertebral foramina in *spondylosis*.

Lumbar spondylosis

This is degeneration of the intervertebral discs in the lumbar region. With age, the discs tend to lose their elasticity and ability to act as shock absorbers and the disc space becomes narrowed. Because the mechanism of the intervertebral joint is disturbed the posterior articulations which are synovial joints may become osteoarthritic. This combination of disc degeneration and secondary osteoarthritis is known as *spondylosis*, although this term is often used to denote simply degeneration of the discs. Osteophyte formation (*see* Osteoarthritis, Chapter 3) around the margins of the vertebral bodies and joints is called 'lipping' and their encroachment into the intervertebral foramina may cause irritation of a nerve root. A patient with spondylosis may have symptoms similar to but usually not so severe as a prolapsed disc.

Lumbar disc prolapse (slipped disc)

Each intervertebral disc consists of a dense ring of fibrous tissue—the annulus fibrosus—which surrounds a soft fluid-like centre—the nucleus pulposus. The main function of the discs is to act as 'shock absorbers' in the vertebral column. Lesions can occur in these discs and problems are most likely to arise in the regions of the spine that are more mobile and also subject to the greatest strains. *Prolapse* of an intervertebral disc is most common in the lower lumbar spine (between L4/5 or L5/S1) and can be an acute event during continuing disc degeneration (*spondylosis*). In disc prolapse the nucleus bulges through a rent in the annulus. If the disc prolapses backwards it may impinge upon the contents of the spinal canal but as the central part of the disc is strengthened posteriorly by the longitudinal ligament, a prolapse directed to one side of this structure is more likely. In this case the prolapse presses on a nerve root and the patient may feel pain—*sciatica*—and experience sensory impairment and weakness in the area supplied by that particular nerve root.

Because intervertebral discs are normally non-opaque to X-rays, plain radiography may be supplemented by contrast studies in the investigation of disc lesions, e.g. in myelography, radiculography and discography. Plain films may, however, give evidence of disc derangement in that the vertebral bodies may be slightly malaligned. Lateral projections taken in flexion and extension may also show instability in the vertebrae caused by this joint defect.

Spondylolisthesis

Spondylolisthesis literally means a slipping vertebra—one slipping forwards on the vertebra below. The condition is most common in the fifth lumbar vertebra and the patient

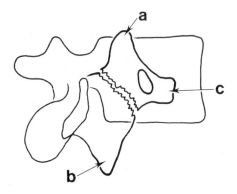

Figure 8.8. The left pars interarticularis defect as would be visible on the left anteroposterior oblique radiograph. For key, *see* text

may be affected by lower back pain and symptoms of nerve root pressure. Most cases of spondylolisthesis occur because of a defect in the lamina (pars interarticularis) of the slipping vertebra.

This defect may be congenital but the majority of these lesions are thought to be attributable to stress fractures of one or both sides of the neural arch through the relatively weak pars interarticularis. This area of a lumbar vertebra is best demonstrated in the oblique projection. In this view the outline of the lamina, superior (*Figure 8.8a*) and inferior (*Figure 8.8b*) articular processes and the transverse process (*Figure 8.8c*) resemble the silhouette of a Scots terrier, the pars interarticularis corresponding to the neck of the dog. A defect appears as a collar on the dog (*Figure 8.9*).

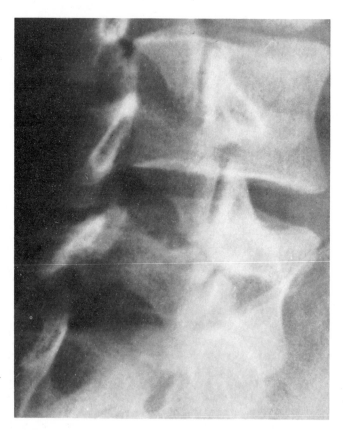

Figure 8.9. Left anteroposterior oblique projection of the lower lumbar spine. A defect is visible through the left pars interarticularis of the fifth lumbar vertebrae

Spondylolysis

This is the presence of a pars interarticularis defect without forward slipping of the vertebra.

Ankylosing spondylitis

See page 146 and Chapter 3.

Lordosis

The normal anteroposterior curve in the lumbar spine is convex in the forwards direction. This is known as the lumbar lordosis. An abnormal increase in this curve can be produced where there is incorrect distribution of the weight of the trunk through the lumbar vertebrae. This has the effect of tiring the muscles of the back and an unsupported spine sags in its most mobile region—the lumbar region. The condition is sometimes called *swayback*.

An increased lordosis may also be the result of compensation for an exaggerated kyphosis in the thoracic spine.

Sacralization and lumbarization

Sacralization is the complete or partial fusion of L5 with S1. In some individuals the transverse process of the fifth lumbar vertebra on one or both sides may be enlarged. Often this enlargement is only slight but in other cases the process may be fused with the sacrum and ilium. The sacralized transverse process may form a false joint—*pseudoarthrosis*.

Lumbarization is where the first sacral segment is not part of the sacrum but anatomically is similar to a lumbar vertebra and is separated from the second sacral segment by a rudimentary intervertebral disc. These two anomalies may be the cause of low back pain.

Lumbosacral facets

The lumbosacral facets may be rotated and asymmetrical. This is another congenital anomaly that predisposes to back pain.

Spina bifida

Incomplete development of the neural arches of the vertebrae such that they are not completely fused posteriorly. This can be simply a small gap in the spinous processes which is bridged by unossified cartilage—*spina bifida occulta*. When the bony defect is more extensive, the contents of the spinal canal may be exposed on the surface—*myelomeningocele*—usually in the lumbar region. In severe forms of spina bifida there may be other abnormalities of the vertebrae and ribs. The patient may also have *hydrocephalus* due to obstruction to the outflow of cerebrospinal fluid from the fourth ventricle by a protrusion of the cerebellum into the foramen magnum—*Arnold–Chiari malformation* (*see* Chapter 10).

If nerve tissue is involved in spina bifida the patient will have functional impairment of the lower limbs and some degree of loss of bowel and bladder control. As a result of muscle imbalance, various lower limb deformities may develop and these may be controlled by the use of splintage and surgical operations.

New growths

In the spine the majority of these are secondary metastatic deposits from a primary—usually a carcinoma of the breast or lung. The tumour may cause collapse of a vertebral body. Primary tumours arising from either the bone or the contents of the spinal canal are quite rare. Tumours of the nerve tissue only infrequently cause changes in the surrounding bony structures and usually have to be investigated by an X-ray examination using a contrast agent such as in myelography.

Thoracic and lumbar spine injuries

Wedge fractures of vertebral bodies

From the dorsal to the upper lumbar region the curve and movement of the spine are predominantly of flexion. If a force acts along the vertical axis of the spine in either direction then the vertebral column will probably *hyperflex*. The anterior portion of one or more vertebral bodies will be compressed. These crush or *wedge fractures* (*Figure 8.10*) are the commonest in the thoracic and thoracolumbar regions of the spine, especially in the osteoporotic bones of the elderly whose bones often need minimal trauma before they are damaged (*see* Chapter 3). Wedge compression fractures tend to heal fairly easily but there may be a residual wedge deformity in the affected bone (*see* also Senile kyphosis, page 138).

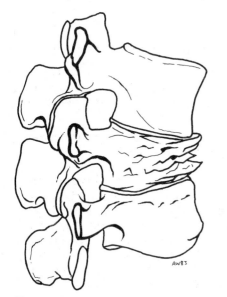

Figure 8.10. A crush or compression fracture of a vertebral body resulting in a wedge-like deformity, sometimes termed a 'wedge' fracture

Fracture–dislocations

In spinal injuries the danger of associated damage to nerve roots and cord is of prime importance and this danger is always greatly increased when fractures of the neural arch permits a fracture dislocation to develop.

Moving down the vertebral column from the thoracic to lumbar regions, the joint facets of the superior and inferior articular processes become more vertically inclined. This makes pure dislocation of the joints almost impossible. A fracture through the articular processes would not necessarily make the spine unstable on movement simply because stability of the spine depends on the integrity of the vertebral body disc joint (anterior joint), the posterior joints (facet joints) and the spinal ligaments. The type of injury required to disrupt all of these components is a forceful flexion and rotation of the spine, e.g. caused by a fall from a height on to the shoulder or a rock fall over a flexed back.

Typically the injury occurs at a level somewhere between T10 and L2 and produces a shearing fracture just below the disc—a *slice fracture* (*Figure 8.11*). The upper vertebral body is displaced forwards on the lower and as the fracture is unstable the patient should be moved carefully, avoiding flexion and rotation of the back. Unfortunately, damage to the contents of the spinal canal is common, so there is a great risk of paraplegia. Complex vertebral fractures can sometimes be investigated using *computerized tomography*.

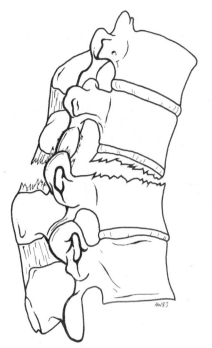

Figure 8.11. Fracture–dislocation in the thoraco-lumbar spine

Transverse process fractures in the lumbar spine

These commonly occur following either a direct injury or a sudden muscle pull—*avulsion fracture*. The fracture virtually always unites without requiring any special treatment. Because there is a risk of renal or other abdominal injury these patients will be admitted for a 48-hour period of observation.

Nerve injuries at different levels of the thoracic and lumbar spines

Injury to the spinal cord and nerve roots is not a guaranteed outcome in fractures of the vertebral column, however the probability of nerve injury occurring varies according to the vertebral level involved:

(1) *Thoracic spine:* a fracture–dislocation usually causes complete transection of the cord. Paraplegia is common.
(2) *Thoracolumbar spine (T12/L1):* the lower segments of the spinal cord and the proximal roots of the cauda equina lie side by side in the spinal canal. A nerve lesion caused by a fracture may be a mixed one. Sometimes the cord may be damaged but not the nerve roots.
(3) *Lumbar spine:* below the level of L1 the vertebral canal contains the cauda equina (level of cord termination does vary) and this structure is more resistant to injury than the cord itself.

The sacrum, sacroiliac joints and the coccyx

Injuries

Fractures of the sacrum

This injury is caused by a fall or direct blow on the sacral region. The fracture is usually no more than a crack but there can be complications if the sacral foramina are involved where nerves may be damaged.

Traumatic dislocation of a sacroiliac joint

In serious pelvic injuries the continuity of the pelvic ring is disrupted in two places. This can be brought about by a fracture of the pelvis both above the level of the hip—usually through the ilium—and below the level of the hip through the pubic bones. The fracture of the ilium may extend into the sacroiliac joint but sometimes widening (diastasis) of a sacroiliac joint may occur (*see* page 163).

Other conditions

Ankylosing spondylitis

The sacroiliac joints are usually the first to be affected in this disease, the bony surfaces undergo a degeneration and the joint space may be widened. Later on the joints may become completely fused—*ankylosis*. The sacroiliac joints may be affected by other inflammatory disease. *See* also Chapter 3.

New growths

The sacrum may be a site for metastatic new growths. A primary carcinoma of the rectum may infiltrate the sacrum which is its close posterior relation.

Congenital abnormalities

There are two congenital defects of the sacrum which although very rare result in a deformity of the pelvic inlet and thus have obstetric importance:

(1) *Naegele's pelvis:* one wing of the sacrum is absent with ankylosis of the sacroiliac joint on the affected side.
(2) *Robert's pelvis:* a bilateral Naegele's pelvis.

Coccydynia

This is pain in the region of the coccyx on sitting, especially on a hard surface; it tends to occur in women, usually after a fall but sometimes after childbirth. Radiographs may show an abnormally long coccyx or acute anterior angulation of it.

Radiographic techniques

Two projections of the specified area taken at right angles to each other are the minimal requirements for an examination of the spine. These are the anteroposterior and lateral projections. Where further information is needed concerning the neural arch, the *posterior* or *apophyseal joints* between the superior and inferior articular processes and the *intervertebral foramina*, oblique projections are taken.

Cervical spine

The positioning is usually undertaken with the patient erect unless the patient's condition precludes this. The position is chosen first for reasons of convenience, and secondly because gravity tends to aid depression of the shoulders—important in the lateral projection (6). It is also customary to use a secondary radiation grid when examining the cervical spine, but this can sometimes be omitted for the lateral projection (6), where the significant air gap 'cleans up' scattered radiation to an acceptable degree.

For planes and lines of reference for positioning of the head in cervical spine techniques refer to Chapter 10.

(1) Anteroposterior C1–C3

To reveal the upper cervical vertebrae the patient must be radiographed with the mouth open. The head must be carefully positioned so that neither teeth, alveolar process of maxillae nor occiput obscure the vertebrae. The patient is supine or erect facing the X-ray tube. The median sagittal plane remains perpendicular to the table and film.

The patient is asked to open the mouth wide and the head is adjusted until the maxillae are felt to be superimposed on the occiput (*Figure 8.12*). The head must be immobilized. The mouth can be held open with a non-opaque bite-block.

Centre—Through the open mouth parallel to a line joining the upper incisors (or hard palate if edentulous) with the lower margin of the occipital bone.

Note—The central ray does not have to be perpendicular to the film. Generally the X-ray tube makes an angle of 20 degrees with the orbitomeatal base line. The important principle is that the beam is tangential to the obscuring bones of the base of skull and face. If the patient cannot open the mouth then only tomography can satisfactorily demonstrate this region in the anteroposterior plane.

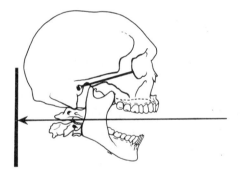

Figure 8.12. The principles of relative patient and X-ray beam positioning in projection (1). The dotted line reperesents the hard palate

(2) Odontoid process

This is demonstrated in the following projections:

   (i) Anteroposterior C1–C3 (projection (1)).
 (ii) Lateral C1–C7 (projection (6)).
(iii) Anteroposterior C1–C7 (projection (5))—moving jaw technique.

Where the patient cannot open the mouth or where visualization in the normal anteroposterior projection is impossible because of a condition such as *platybasia* alternative projections can be taken:

(iv) *Anteroposterior axial:* the patient is supine or erect. The median sagittal plane is perpendicular to the film. The orbitomeatal base line is raised to be 45 degrees to the film.

Centre: at a point midway between the external auditory meatus (EAMs) with the X-ray tube angled 35 degrees cephalad.

(v) *Posteroanterior axial:* the patient is prone or erect. The medial sagittal plane is perpendicular to the film. The orbitomeatal base line is raised to be 45 degrees to the film.

Centre: midway between the EAMs with the X-ray tube angled 30 degrees caudad.

The process is also demonstrated in the following:

(vi) Lateral for atlanto-occipital joints [projection (3(ii))].

(vii) Anteroposterior obliques for atlanto-occipital joints [projection (3(iv))].

(viii) Submentovertical skull (projection (7), page 184).

There may be doubt over the presence of a fracture of the process. This could be due to artefactual shadows. A common example is the cleft between the two upper incisor teeth which can be 'projected' on to the process in projection (1) and be mistaken for a vertical splint. (The peg nearly always fractures transversely across its base.) If this occurs at the initial examination then a second anteroposterior projection (1) could be taken with the X-ray tube at a slightly different angle.

(ix) Because of the problems associated with plain radiography of the area, the odontoid process is a good candidate for *tomography* and *autotomography* (*see* page 186).

(3) Atlas and atlanto-occipital joints

(i) *Anteroposterior C1–C3 (projection (1))*—The atlas and especially its joints with the skull are more easily shown in the anteroposterior aspect if the patient has no teeth.

(ii) *Lateral atlanto-occipital joints*—The median sagittal plane is parallel to the cassette and grid. *Centre:* 2.5 cm below the EAM with the X-ray beam perpendicular to the film. The joints are overshadowed by the mastoid processes of the temporal bone in the lateral projection.

(iii) *Posteroanterior atlanto-occipital joints*—The patient is erect or prone facing the bucky table. The orbitomeatal base line is perpendicular to the film and the median sagittal plane is perpendicular to the film. *Centre:* 2.5 cm below the external occipital protruberance with a 'straight' X-ray beam. Both joints are projected through the maxillary antra.

(iv) *Anteroposterior oblique atlanto-occipital joints*—The patient is supine or erect facing the X-ray tube. The orbitomeatal base line is 90 degrees to the film and the median sagittal plane is perpendicular to the film. *Centre:* so the X-ray beam is midway between the orbits. Then rotate the head to the left so the central ray is *over* the right orbit—this will demonstrate the right joint. Repeat for the other side, rotating the head to the right so the central ray is over the left orbit. Where injury is suspected to the upper cervical spine movement of the head should not be deliberately sought until permission is granted by the radiologist or casualty officer.

(v) *Tomography* may be required in the anteroposterior and lateral positions.

Posterior arch of atlas

(vi) *Anteroposterior C1–C3 (projection (1))*—This may show any lateral displacement if a fracture is present.

(vii) *A lateral projection* can be taken as for projection (3(ii)), centring over the joints but with the X-ray tube angled 20 degrees cephalad.

(viii) *Submentovertical skull* (projection (7), page 184), if permissible.

(4) Anteroposterior C3–C7

The patient is supine or erect facing the X-ray tube. The median sagittal plane is perpendicular to the film. Raise the chin slightly so that the orbitomeatal base line makes an angle of 70 degrees with the film.

The aim of the positioning is to reveal the maximum number of cervical vertebrae and the disc spaces. The jaw or occiput will usually obscure the upper two vertebrae in this projection.

Centre—To the sternal notch then angle the beam 10 degrees cephalad; *or* with a 'straight' X-ray beam over the sternal notch open the collimators so the beam will include C3 (*Figure 8.13*). Use lead protection over the sternal area.

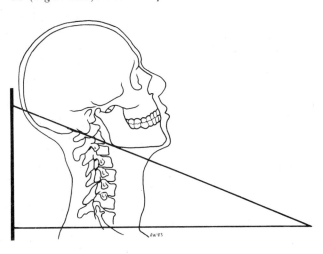

Figure 8.13. Patient positioning in projection (4). With the X-ray tube centred over the sternal notch the lower border of the mandible and occiput become superimposed on the film with the X-ray tube perpendicular to the film and centred over the sternal notch

The oblique rays in either case should project the lower border of the jaw over the occiput.

Hyperextension of neck, patient with 'short' neck

A curved cassette can be used which reduces subject–film distance. The advantage of using a secondary radiation grid is now lost. The occiput may also obscure more of the upper vertebra; a caudal angulation of the X-ray beam may help to reduce this effect.

Neck held in flexion

Where the patient cannot raise the chin adequately an additional cephalad tube angulation can be made to project the jaw upwards away from the spine.

Torticollis

With the patient supine it may sometimes be possible to assist the patient *gently* to straighten the rotation of the head. Otherwise the anteroposterior projection will have to be taken in whatever position the patient can manage.

Cervical rib

A collimated view can also be taken of the area. Position as for projection (4).
    Centre—Over the sternal notch with the X-ray tube angled 15 degrees cephalad.

(5) Anteroposterior C1–C7 (moving jaw)

This technique can be used as an alternative to projections (1) and (4). Position the head as for projection (1) and immobilize it adequately. Ask the patient to open and close the mouth gently and slowly in a continuous fashion. Rehearse this before making the exposure.
    Centre—To the lower tip of the symphysis menti. Use a long exposure time, e.g. 4 seconds. The mouth movement during the exposure causes the jaw image to be diffused over the cervical spine. (The head must not be allowed to move otherwise the image of the spine will become blurred.)

(6) Lateral C1–C7

The patient sits in the general lateral position with the affected side (if relevant) nearest the film. The shoulder touches the bucky or cassette. The median sagittal plane is parallel to the film and the chin is raised slightly to move the jaw angle away from the vertebrae. The lower border of the cassette must be at shoulder level and the shoulders depressed as far as possible so that C7 is included on the film.

Centre—2.5 cm behind the angle of the jaw over C3 with a horizontal X-ray beam. The focal–film distance is increased to 150 cm because of the large subject–film distance. (Alternative technique—projection (7).) Where difficulty in demonstrating C7 is experienced refer to the techniques for the cervicothoracic region (projections (12–16)).

(7) Where the patient must be examined in a horizontal position

The patient is supine. The shoulders are equidistant from the table top. A cassette is propped vertically alongside the patient's neck, its lower border lying below the level of the shoulder. The head and neck are adjusted so that the median sagittal plane is perpendicular to the film. An assistant (not a radiographer) given radiation protection can pull gently downwards on the patient's arms so that the lower cervical vertebrae are shown on the film.

Centre—As for projection (6).

Torticollis

An initial film should be positioned on the side *away* from the tilted neck and a horizontal beam centred just above the shoulder nearest the X-ray tube. Immobilization may be aided if the patient is supine. More than one lateral projection may be required in order to demonstrate all the cervical vertebrae.

Injuries

Patients with suspected bony injury to the neck are likely to be brought to the department on a stretcher. The greatest care should be taken if an orthopaedic collar or other such support needs to be removed. The general rule is always to seek medical advice or assistance.

The lateral projection (7) should be taken first and inspected before any further movement of the head and neck are permitted.

Patient on traction

Where continuous traction is used as a method of treatment for dislocation or subluxation of the vertebrae the radiographer will be required to take a lateral film at intervals during the treatment. The examination is undertaken on the ward or in the intensive care unit.

(8) Lateral obliques for articular facets ('Lodge–Moor' obliques)

In injuries the conventional lateral projection (7) may not adequately demonstrate the relationship between the articular facets. Using 'Lodge–Moor' obliques the apophyseal joints are shown in profile.

Two films are taken with the patient rotated 20 degrees from the supine position towards each side in turn (*Figure 8.14*). The raised shoulder is supported. The cassette is

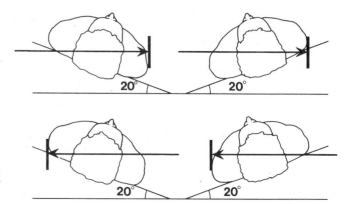

Figure 8.14. Positioning of patient, film and direction of the X-ray beam for the Lodge–Moor oblique projections

propped in the same position as in projection (7). Traction is maintained on the arms. A further two films are taken with the X-ray tube directed from the *other* side of the patient.

Centre—To C5 (thyroid cartilage) with a horizontal beam. When the raised side is nearest the X-ray tube, angle the tube 5 degrees cephalad. When the raised side is away from the X-ray tube, angle the tube 5 degrees caudad. FFD is 122 cm. Where the patient cannot be moved use projection (11).

(9) Laterals in flexion and extension

These will show changes in alignment of the cervical vertebrae in cases of instability caused by injury. They should not be undertaken at an initial examination unless under medical sanction and supervision. Flexion and extension views can be carried out later during treatment management to confirm that the spine is stable.

(10) Anteroposterior obliques for intervertebral foramina

The patient sits on a rotating stool with his back to the vertical bucky. Rotate the patient's whole body through 45 degrees towards one side. Continue turning the head until the median sagittal plane of the head is parallel to the film. Raise the chin slightly.

Centre—Over the sternomastoid muscle at mid-neck level of the side nearest the tube with a horizontal beam. Angulation of the X-ray tube upwards (e.g. by 15 degrees) may improve visualization of the foramina especially where the cervical lordosis is exaggerated. Focal–film distance is 150 cm. Repeat for the other side. The foramina demonstrated are on the side of the neck *nearest* the X-ray tube.

These 45 degree obliques may be done in the posteroanterior position, in which case the foramina demonstrated are on the side nearest the film.

(11) Alternative technique

Where obliques are required but the patient cannot be moved from the supine position: the X-ray beam is angled transversely across the patient's neck making an angle of 45 degrees with the median sagittal plane.

Centre—5 cm lateral to and at the level of the thyroid eminence. Care must be taken when the casette is placed under the patient's head and neck. Ensure that the spine cannot be 'projected off' the film.

Cervicothoracic spine

(12) Anteroposterior

Position as for projection (4).

Centre—To the sternal notch, lowering the film to include the relevant vertebrae.

This region of the vertebral column is largely obscured by the shoulders in the lateral aspect. Failure to produce a lateral or alternative projection in cases of injury may result in an abnormality being missed. This is of special significance in the lower cervical spine where injury is more likely to occur but can often be inadequately demonstrated when only conventional lateral views are taken (6 or 7).

Projection (13) usually reveals no further down than C7. Projections (14–16) are alternative methods for demonstrating the lower cervical and upper thoracic spine. Further information can be obtained by using tomography.

(13) Lateral

Position and centre as for projection (6). Sandbags are held in each hand to aid depression of the shoulders. In most patients C7 will be shown. The exposure can be increased from projection (6).

(14) Lateral oblique

More suitable for the broad-shouldered patient. With the patient sitting in the lateral position the side nearest the

X-ray tube is rotated backwards through 20 degrees. The arm nearest the support is moved forwards, the other arm backwards.

Centre—With a horizontal beam just below the mid-point of the clavicle furthest from the film.

The spine is visualized between the shoulders. A large exposure is required for this projection. Because of the steep range of subject density present, the cervicothoracic region is a good candidate for *high kilovoltage technique*.

Projection (15)

The patient sits in the lateral position. The arm nearest the film is folded over the head. The posterior aspect of the raised arm and the axilla touch the bucky. The other arm lies in internal rotation along the side of the trunk, this shoulder being depressed as far as possible.

Centre—With a horizontal X-ray beam just above the shoulder nearest the X-ray tube to pass through the axilla nearest the film.

Projection (16)

The patient stands in the lateral position next to the vertical bucky. The neck is flexed forwards and the arms brought downwards and folded across the chest. The aim is to bring the shoulders in front of the spine.

Centre—With a horizontal beam, just above the head of the humerus remote from the film.

Spinous processes

Use either a high kilovoltage technique or multiple radiography to demonstrate spinous processes as well as the vertebral bodies.

Thoracic spine

(17) Anteroposterior thoracic spine

The patient is supine with the arms by the sides. The shoulders and anterior superior iliac spines of the pelvis are equidistant from the table top. The head should be supported on a pad or pillow.

Centre—2.5 cm below the sternal angle with a vertical beam.

Expose on deep arrested inspiration. The variance in physical density of the overlying structures—trachea, heart and diaphragm—may make it necessary for separate films to be exposed to demonstrate adequately all of the thoracic vertebrae.

(18) Lateral (T3–T12)

The patient lies on the affected side with his back to the radiographer. Flex the patient's hips and knees for support. Raise both arms over the head, placing the lower arm under the pillow. The long axis of the vertebrae should be parallel to the film and perpendicular to the central ray if the disc joint spaces are to be demonstrated. Adjust the position with non-opaque pads. The surface of the patient's back should be seen to be perpendicular to the table top, i.e. rotation must be avoided. Check that the ilia and shoulders are superimposed.

Centre—Over T6.

Expose on deep arrested inspiration; *or* if the patient's thorax is immobilized with a broad bucky band a long exposure time can be used with the patient breathing gently to produce diffusion of lung markings and ribs over the vertebrae.

In the lower thoracic region there is an abrupt change in subject density due to the transition from over-shadowing by lung to diaphragm. Quite often a second localized lateral projection must be taken on arrested expiration with relevant exposure change to show T12. The lateral can also be taken in the erect position, i.e. weight bearing.

(19) Anteroposterior obliques

These projections are used for further information about the rib or intervertebral articulations. From the anteroposterior position the patient is rotated 45 degrees to either side and supported.

Centre—In the mid-clavicular line of the raised side, 5 cm below the level of the sternal angle.

Kyphosis and kyphos

Where there is a generalized increase in spinal curvature supine positioning for the anteroposterior projection may be acceptable. To prevent discomfort non-opaque pads should be placed under the patient to give adequate support. Where a sharp angulation is present (possibly due to more acute pathology) or where the patient would suffer discomfort in lying on his back, erect positioning may be preferable.

Centre—To the apex of the spinal curve (*Figure 8.15*). In extreme cases it may be difficult to produce a good anteroposterior view and more than one film may be required with appropriate tube angulation.

Note that the lateral projection may require a lot less exposure than the anteroposterior because the vertebrae may be very prominent.

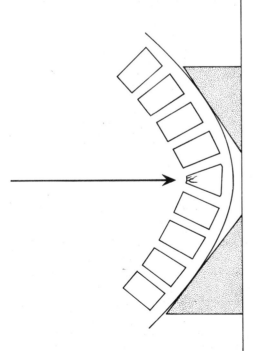

Figure 8.15. Centring the X-ray beam to the apex of the spinal curve in kyphosis

Scoliosis

At the initial examination radiographs taken will probably include erect and supine anteroposterior and lateral views of the spine from the occiput to the sacrum. A special cassette is used which is both long and wide enough to accommodate the whole spine.

Anteroposterior projections may also be taken with the patient 'side-bending'. These determine flexibility of the spine and indicate how much each curve corrects passively. Side-bending films help to distinguish structural from non-structural curves.

'Bone age' can be checked by reference to the state of the iliac crest epiphyses and by determining bone age which has importance in the planning of treatment.

From the spine films, abnormal curves will be assessed and measured. Comparisons will be made with radiographs taken before and during treatments.

Injuries

In more serious spinal trauma two projections must be taken *without* moving the patient. Use of a casualty table system is preferable. The anteroposterior projection *must* be adequately exposed if a fracture is suspected in the thoracolumbar region. If the patient must remain prone then a posteroanterior projection must suffice. It may not be possible to adjust the patient's position if he is rotated.

The patient's arms are raised, and a lateral is taken with a horizontal X-ray beam. The cassette and grid are propped alongside the patient's chest. The spine may be partially obscured by the mattress shadow if the patient is supine. There is little that can be done about this but major bony displacements should be visible. The film level and exposure should be adjusted if both thoracic and lumbar spines are to be shown.

Lumbar spine

Use of radiation protection is important at the lower vertebral levels. In special circumstances abdominal preparation may be required.

(20) Anteroposterior L1–L5

The patient is supine with the arms by the sides. The shoulders and anterior superior iliac spines are equidistant from the table top. Either the legs are outstretched *or* the hips and knees are flexed in order to flatten the lumbar lordosis.

Centre—In the mid-line at the level of the lower costal margin (over L3). Expose on arrested expiration *or* using a long exposure time the patient breathes quietly to produce diffusion of bowel shadows over the spine. The film should show soft-tissue outlines of the psoas muscle and kidney on either side of the spine.

Alternative technique—projection (21).

Transverse processes

The exposure should be reduced where necessary.

Weight bearing

Changes in vertebral alignment can be seen if the anteroposterior projection is taken in the erect position.

(21) Posteroanterior L1–L5

In the prone position the divergent rays pass more directly through the vertebral body joint spaces as the spine's convexity is towards the film.

Centre—As for projection (20).

Check that the patient is not rotated. The upper chest and lower legs should be supported on pillows.

(22) Anteroposterior L5–S1 joint space

Using the same position as in projection (20). The X-ray tube is angled cephalad between 5 and 25 degrees so that the central ray passes through the joint space (*Figure 8.16*). Degree of angulation depends on the lumbosacral angle.

Centre—In the mid-line at the level of the anterior superior iliac spines.

Alternatively, the patient can be prone as in projection (21).

Centre—To the fifth lumbar spinous process with the X-ray tube angled 5–15 degrees caudally.

Collimate the beam in either position. The cassette must be sufficiently displaced in alignment with the beam.

(23) Lateral L1–S1

The patient lies on the affected side or with his back to the radiographer. The knees and hips are flexed for support. The position is adjusted so the ilia and shoulders are superimposed. The trunk must not be rotated. The long axis of the spine should be parallel to the film and perpendicular to the central ray (*Figures 8.17 and 8.18*). This can be achieved by placing non-opaque pads under the chest, waist and between the legs. Compensatory tube angulation may also be needed.

Centre—Over the body of L3 at the level of the lower costal margin. Exposed on arrested expiration.

Place a piece of lead rubber on the table top just behind

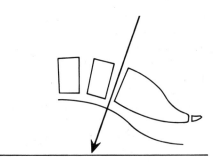

Figure 8.16. The central ray, angulated upwards to pass through the joint space between the body of L5 and the sacrum in projection (22)

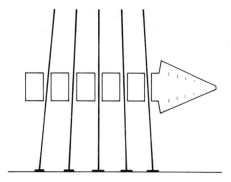

Figure 8.17. The spine positioned with its long axis parallel to the film in projection (23). The X-ray beam passes through the vertebral body joint spaces and these are clearly demonstrated on the resultant film

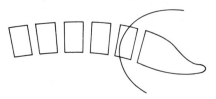

Figure 8.18. Outline appearance of the lumbar vertebral bodies and their joint spaces as seen on the lateral lumbar spine radiograph in projection (23)

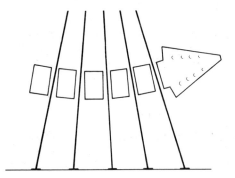

Figure 8.19. Placing a patient with lumbar scoliosis in projection (23)

the patient's back. This will prevent scattered radiation produced in the subject from reaching the film and affecting the image. If the patient has a lumbar scoliosis (*Figure 8.19*), position him so that the convexity of the curve is directed towards the film.

Spinous processes

The processes are frequently collimated off or over-exposed on routine films. A lateral projection with reduced kilovoltage may be required.

(24) *Lateral L5–S1 joint space*

Quite often this area is inadequately demonstrated on projection (23) because it requires a rather larger exposure than the rest of the lumbar spine. The patient remains in the same position and the direction of the L5–S1 body joint space is assessed by palpating the dimples next to the posterior superior iliac spines. The central ray should pass directly through the space so a tube angulation may be needed.

Centre—With a collimated beam 7.5 cm in front of the spinous process of L5.

A much higher kilovoltage may be needed to penetrate the mass of bone in the lateral position. Often the state or angle of the joint can be determined by looking at the anteroposterior L1–L5 film. Where repeated attempts at producing a joint space fail, the radiographer should repeat the film but with the patient lying on the *other* side. If the fifth lumbar vertebra is *sacralized* a joint space cannot be shown.

(25) *Laterals in flexion and extension*

Demonstrates any *instability* of the spine by showing changes in alignment of the bodies. The patient is erect in the lateral position with one side touching the vertical bucky.

Instruct the patient to bend forwards and then backwards and take a film in each position. The patient can rest the tips of his fingers (for security) on a chair placed first in front and then behind him.

The film should be large enough to include the lumbosacral region or the entire lumbar spine as necessary. A broad bucky band may help immobilization but may be difficult to use in this situation.

Bone grafts

Some surgeons treated *spondylolisthesis* by grafting bone across the spinous processes (posterior fusion). Where this is done the graft should be demonstrated on the radiograph—a reduced kilovoltage or other exposure manipulation may be needed.

Normal posture

An erect lateral can be taken with the patient simply standing 'straight' as they would do normally.

(26) Anteroposterior obliques lumbar spine

From the supine position the patient is rotated to one side between 25 and 35 degrees and supported.

Centre—At the level of the lower costal margin over the mid-clavicular line of the raised side. Repeat raising the opposite side. The pars interarticularis and facet joints on the side nearest the film are shown. If L5–S1 is the area of interest in *spondylolisthesis* then the centring point may be lowered.

Injuries

For major injuries the same comments apply as for the thoracic spine (*see* page 156).

Sacrum, sacroiliac joints, coccyx

Non-urgent cases for examination may have abdominal preparation as this region of the spine is frequently obscured by bowel shadows. The '10-day rule' should be adhered to.

(27) Anteroposterior sacrum and coccyx

The patient is supine with the legs extended and both knees rest on a pillow. The anterior superior iliac spines are equidistant from the table top. Use gonad protection for males.

For the sacrum

Centre—In the mid-line above the symphysis pubis with the X-ray tube angled between 5 and 15 degrees cephalad. Because of the lumbosacral lordosis the anterior surface of the sacrum faces both forwards and downwards when the patient is supine. To produce an undistorted image the beam must be at 90 degrees to the sacral long axis. The cephalad tube angle required increases for females.

For the coccyx

Centre—In the mid-line 5 cm above the symphysis pubis.

The beam is angled 15 degrees caudally to separate the coccyx and symphysis.

Injuries

If the patient cannot lie on his back but can stand, these projections can be taken in the erect position. Attempt to flatten the lumbar lordosis against the bucky table.

(28) Lateral sacrum and coccyx

Position as for projection (23). The median sagittal plane of the pelvis should be parallel to the film.

For the sacrum

Centre—7.5 cm anterior to the skin surface, over the posterior superior iliac spines. This distance will vary according to the thickness of soft tissues.

A relatively large kilovoltage is required to penetrate the density of bone. The beam should be collimated and lead rubber placed on the table top surface as in projection (23). (In most patients the coccyx is superficial and will be over-exposed in this projection.)

For the coccyx

Centre—To the coccyx which lies between the buttocks. Accurate centring is needed otherwise the subject will be projected off the film (owing to the large subject–film distance). The exposure can be substantially reduced.

(29) Sacroiliac joints

(i) Oblique projection

The joint surfaces lie in an anteroposterior and lateromedial direction as they pass from the front to the back of the posterior pelvic wall. For a relatively clear visualization of the joint space the side of interest must be raised (from the supine position) until the joint is perpendicular to the film (*Figure 8.20*).

Centre—2.5 cm medial to the anterior superior iliac spine of the raised side. The X-ray tube may be angled cephalad 5–15 degrees according to the angle of the sacrum (*see* projection (27)). Repeat for the other side.

(ii) Anteroposterior

Position and centre the patient as for projection (27, sacrum). The tube angulation is 10–25 degrees cephalad. Both sacroiliac joints are demonstrated.

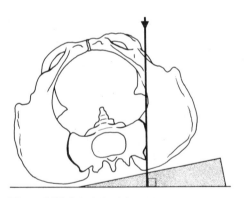

Figure 8.20. Principle of the patient positioning and direction of the central ray in projection (29)

(iii) Posteroanterior

This is an alternative projection to (29(ii)) and is often favoured because the diverging rays pass through the joint spaces. The patient is prone with a pillow placed under the ankles. Check that there is no rotation of the pelvis.

Centre—In the mid-line at the level of the dimples over the posterior superior iliac spines. The tube is angled 5–15 degrees caudally.

Further information about the joints can be obtained using *tomography*.

Subluxation

Two erect anteroposterior views are taken with the patient weight bearing on alternate feet (*see* Instability of the symphysis, page 166).

9 The pelvis: the innominate bones

The pelvic girdle is formed by the two innominate bones which are joined anteriorly by a symphysis. Posteriorly the two ilia (wings) are separated by the wedge-shaped sacrum which forms the paired sacroiliac joints.

The ring-like structure of the pelvis has two basic functions—to support the abdominal contents and to transmit the forces of weight bearing from the spine to the lower limbs.

The term pelvis means basin. Anatomically it can be divided into two segments—the upper, wider false pelvis and the lower, narrow true pelvis.

The characteristic differences between the male and the female pelvis have been the subject of much study for use in the fields of forensic science and anthropology. In obstetrics the measurements of the true pelvis are of great significance and can be assessed, where necessary, by the radiographic technique of *pelvimetry*.

Anatomically the sacrum and coccyx form part of the vertebral column and are discussed in Chapter 8.

Indications for the X-ray examination

Injuries

Isolated fractures of the pelvis

A single fracture may occur through the ilium or pubic ramus. This is usually caused by a direct blow and occurs rather more readily in the osteoporotic bones of the elderly.

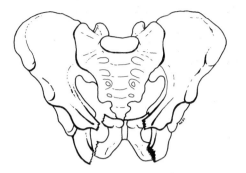

Figure 9.1. Fracture involving all four pubic rami

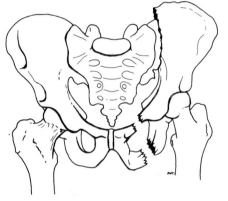

Figure 9.2. Disruption of the pelvic ring by a double fracture through the left ilium and both pubic rami on the same side

Double fractures of the pelvis

This is a much more serious injury where the continuity of the bony circle is broken. There are two major forms:

(1) The anterior portion of the ring may be disrupted if all four pubic rami are broken; the loose portion is driven backwards (*Figure 9.1*).

(2) The pelvic ring is disrupted in two places one of which is above the level of the hip, e.g. a vertical fracture through the ilium from crest to sciatic notch (*Figure 9.2*) or there may be a widening (diastasis) of the sacroiliac joint. Below, either the pubic symphysis is widened or both pubic rami on one side are fractured. Various combinations of these are possible. There may be separation and displacement of fragments.

Double fractures of the pelvis are often complicated by injury to pelvic blood vessels and viscera. Injury to the bladder and urethra are common because the lower ureters, bladder and urethra are closely related to the pelvis. The membranous part of the urethra is the most vulnerable part of the tract in the male. *Cystography* may be used in investigations of bladder injuries.

The rectum is usually only involved in more severe pelvic fractures in which case radiographically there may be fractures through the sacrum and coccyx and gas shadows outside the rectum may also be visible on the films. The internal iliac artery is the main vessel involved in injuries of the pelvis; massive blood loss can occur and the patient may need large transfusions. Because of the serious nature of these complications, their treatment may take precedence over that of the bony injuries.

Fractures of the acetabulum

See Chapter 7.

Other conditions

Paget's disease

The pelvis is one of the bones commonly affected by Paget's disease. It may affect the pubis, ischium or ilium but sometimes only one side of the pelvis is involved. If the disease affects the acetabulum the hip joint may degenerate in a *secondary osteoarthritis* (*see* Chapter 3).

New growths

The pelvis may be affected by metastases from a primary tumour. A carcinoma of the prostate, for example, may spread via the bloodstream to the pubic bones.

Osteitis pubis

This is inflammation of the pubis, which is rare, but may occur after an operation on the bladder or prostate gland. The radiograph may show areas of sclerosis, bone destruction or both.

Extrophy of the bladder

This is a rare congenital condition which involves the musculoskeletal structures of the lower abdomen and the genitourinary tract. There is a wide separation of the pubic bones, sometimes in association with rotational deformities of the pelvic bones around the sacroiliac joints.

Instability of the symphysis pubis

This condition is sometimes observed in professional athletes. In women it may be the result of prolonged parturitional stress. The instability may be the cause of chronic groin pain.

Radiographic techniques

Routinely only one projection is taken of the pelvis (1). In non-urgent cases bowel preparation may sometimes be necessary and the '10-day rule' is adhered to; however, gonad protection in females is not feasible and in males should be used with care.

(1) Anteroposterior pelvis

The patient is supine with the arms folded across the chest. Both legs are extended and placed together and the positioning of the feet is symmetrical (*see* projection (29), page 128). A pillow can be placed under the patient's knees for comfort. The pelvis must be symmetrical—the anterior superior iliac spines must be positioned so that they are equidistant from the table top. The position of the patient's legs can be used as a guide to any degree of rotation present. Correct the pelvis position using non-opaque pads.

Centre—With a vertical beam, between the level of the anterior superior iliac spines and the upper border of the symphysis pubis in the mid-line.

The whole pelvis must be included on the film. If the patient is emaciated then the iliac bones may be over-exposed so a second film may have to be taken. If the patient is of thin physique then the exposure may be made using only a cassette without a grid.

Injuries

It may not be possible to be fussy about the positioning of the pelvis where the patient has serious injuries. Careful attempts should be made to place the patient in the standard position, but the degree of movement tolerated by the patient depends on the extent of injuries elsewhere.

Serious fractures of the pelvic ring are nearly always caused by a crushing force and requests are also likely to be made for radiography of the abdomen and chest. Laterals of both abdomen and chest taken with a horizontal X-ray beam may show free gas in the peritoneal cavity from ruptured bowel and a lateral of the pelvis may also demonstrate a fracture of the sacrum or coccyx.

(2) Lateral pelvis

With the patient remaining in the supine position, a cassette and grid is supported vertically at the side of the patient's pelvis.

Centre—8 cm posterior to the anterior superior iliac spine of the side nearest the X-ray tube using a horizontal beam.

There is a tendency for the patient's sacrum and coccyx to sink into the mattress and thus be obscured by artefacts on the radiograph. Another problem is that this area may be projected off the bottom of the film. To avoid this second situation, the cassette should be positioned so that its lower border is slightly below the level of the table top. A special film holder can be used for this purpose. To reduce magnification of the subject, position the patient as close to the cassette as possible.

Supplementary techniques (3–5 and 6(ii)) should not be attempted with a badly injured patient.

(3) Iliac fossa, ischium and iliac spines

The patient is rotated through 35–45 degrees from the supine position, on to the affected side. The wing of the ilium is now parallel to the film. Support the raised side.

Centre—With a vertical X-ray beam, over the iliac fossa, half way between the anterior superior iliac spine and the mid-line of the pelvis.

(4) Posterior surface of the ilium

From the supine position the affected side is raised until the pelvis has been rotated through 45 degrees. The posterior surface of the ilium of the raised side is now in profile. Support the raised side.

Centre—2.5 cm behind the anterior superior iliac spine of the raised side.

Increase the focal–film distance to 120 cm to compensate for the larger subject–film distance.

(5) Acetabulum

This is demonstrated in the following projections:

  (i) The anteroposterior pelvis (1).
 (ii) The anteroposterior and lateral hip projections (*see* projections (28–35), pages 128–130).
(iii) The projection for the posterior surface of the ilium (4), where both acetabuli are shown.
 (iv) *Profile projection*—From the supine position the pelvis is tilted so the affected side is raised and supported. A cassette and grid are positioned vertically behind the gluteal area of the raised side so that it stands parallel to the neck of the femur. A horizontal X-ray beam is directed so that it is perpendicular to the film.
      Centre: to the head of the femur.
  (v) *'En face' projection*—With the patient prone raise the unaffected side; the body and thighs are maintained at an angle of 45 degrees by non-opaque pads. The acetabulum closest to the table is now approximately parallel to the film.
      Centre: just distal to the coccyx with the X-ray tube angled 12 degrees cephalad. Repeat for the other side.
 (vi) *Tomography and computerized tomography*—For example in complex acetabular fractures.

(6) Pubic bones and pubic symphysis

Localized projections:

 (i) Position the patient as for projection (1): centre over the symphysis with a vertical collimated X-ray beam.
(ii) *Profile projection*—From a sitting position, legs extended, the patient reclines backwards through 30 degrees and is supported. The patient's back makes an angle of 60 degrees with the table. The pubic symphysis is now perpendicular to the film.
     Centre: with a vertical beam over the symphysis pubis.

Instability of the symphysis

The patient stands with her back against the vertical bucky. Position otherwise as for projection (1). Two exposures are made, with the patient taking the full body weight on each leg in turn (so-called 'flamingo views').

Centre—To the symphysis pubis with a horizontal beam. This examination can be done in the posteroanterior position.

10   The skull: cranium and temporal bones

The term 'skull' is intended to refer to the bones of the cranium excluding the facial skeleton. The temporal bones are considered separately because of their complexity.

Indications for the X-ray examination

The cranium (*Figure 10.1*)

This is the box-like structure that encloses the brain and its membranes. It can be arbitrarily divided into the *vault* (lid) and the *base*.

The bones forming the vault are thin, plate-like structures each having a compact bony inner and outer *table* separated by marrow-filled diploë. These bones include mainly the frontal, parietal and occipital bones. The bottom or base of the cranial box is formed by several bones.

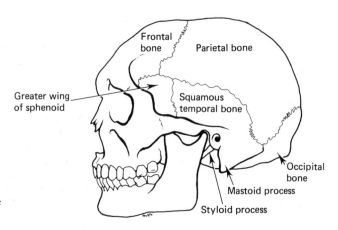

Figure 10.1. Lateral aspect of the skeleton of the head showing the bones of the cranium

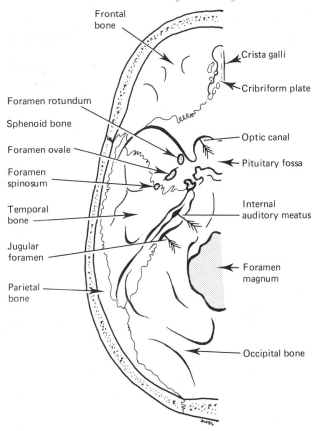

Frontal bone

Crista galli

Cribriform plate

Foramen rotundum

Sphenoid bone

Optic canal

Foramen ovale

Pituitary fossa

Foramen spinosum

Temporal bone

Internal auditory meatus

Jugular foramen

Foramen magnum

Parietal bone

Occipital bone

Figure 10.2. Diagram of the left internal base of the cranium

Starting anteriorly there is the frontal bone forming the roof of the orbits and behind this the 'bird-shaped' sphenoid with its outstretched 'wings'. Lying between the sphenoid and the occiput are the bilateral wedges of the temporal bones. The base of the cranium (*Figure 10.2*), especially in its mid-section, is perforated by the *foramina* which transmit the cranial nerves and blood vessels.

Head injuries

The head can be divided into three main regions when considering injuries—the cranium, the facial bones and the mandible.

The term head injury, however, tends to be used in the situation where there has been trauma to the bones of the cranium and more importantly to the contents of the cranium—the brain.

Apparently there is no strong correlation between a fracture of the skull and the symptoms (or complications) experienced by the patient. Thus a patient may suffer a severe head injury but no bony injury. On the other hand, extensive fractures of the skull may be present with relatively little brain damage.

Head injuries, whether mild or more serious, are relatively common and could constitute about 10% of all new cases referred for radiography in an accident and emergency unit. It has also become common practice for every suspected head injury to be radiographed. The reason for this seems to be mainly medicolegal, and it has been estimated that as many as 44% of all skull X-ray requests are made on these grounds[1].

Mechanism of brain injury

The brain floats in a fluid-filled cavity with little freedom of movement. A blow to the head produces a sudden acceleration (or deceleration) of the skull which the brain does not initially share and so the brain strikes the internal surfaces of the skull contusing (bruising) or lacerating itself on internal projections.

In man, the brain stem joins the cerebrum at right angles so acceleration or deceleration tends to rotate the cerebrum around its junction with the midbrain thus stretching the structures running through this junction. Of these structures the most susceptible is a group of synapses that maintain consciousness—the reticular formation. Traction on these synapses may interrupt conduction, hence the patient may suffer loss of consciousness for a period that varies from seconds to months.

Haemorrhage inside the cranium

This occurs to some degree in all but very minor head injuries but it is significant only if severe enough to produce a *space-occupying clot—a haematoma*.

Haematomas can occur anywhere inside the cranium and are usually classified according to their anatomical site. They may be *intracerebral*, located for example in a ventricle, or they may lie outside the brain between the surrounding layers of meninges. The *extradural haematoma* lies in the potential space between the dura mater and skull whereas a *subdural* haematoma lies in the potential space between the dura and arachnoid membranes. (Various combinations are possible.) The source of these collections of blood can be a torn meningeal or cerebral artery. Alternatively the haemorrhage could originate from a vein or venous sinus.

Whatever the case, this expanding mass presses on the brain (*Figure 10.3*). The cerebral hemisphere of the affected side is pushed away from the haematoma. This can cause a shift in the mid-line structures of the brain which may possibly be detected on the plain anteroposterior radiographs as a shift in the calcified pineal gland (which is calcified in about 30% of adults).

As the volume above the tentorium increases, the medial temporal lobes are pushed further down through the tentorial opening, finally becoming impacted there and

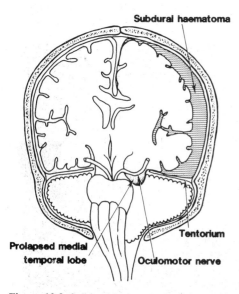

Figure 10.3. Subdural haematoma and its effects

Subdural haematoma

Prolapsed medial temporal lobe

Tentorium

Oculomotor nerve

compressing the midbrain. This is called tentorial herniation of the temporal lobe (pressure cone). The patient can be observed for certain signs. The first of these is a deterioration of the conscious state as the midbrain reticular formation is compressed. Interference with the oculomotor nerve (3rd cranial nerve) may cause changes in the pupil's size and its ability to react to light. The patient is observed for these signs which are recorded on a 'head-injuries' chart.

The pressure of the herniation is now transmitted into the posterior fossa of the skull where the cerebellum and structures of the brain stem are forced downwards into the spinal canal. Compression of vital brain centres during 'coning' is often fatal. Haematomas are investigated and treated by opening the cranium—*craniotomy*—or in the operative procedure of *burr holes*.

Fractures of the skull and their complications

Fractures of the skull have a tendency to occur through the 'weakest' areas of bone. The squamous part of the temporal bone, for instance, is particularly vulnerable because even in adults it may have little more than egg-shell thickness. Fractures have been classified as (1) linear, (2) stellate and (3) depressed.

(1) *Linear fractures*—Most of the fractures of the skull vault are of this kind and in most cases are easy to identify especially when the X-ray beam passes vertically through the fracture (*Figure 10.4*). They appear as sharp, straight radiolucent hair-like lines but they must not be confused with normal vascular markings or suture lines. The majority occur in the parietal region of the vault and may extend down through the squamous portion of the temporal bone to involve the base of the skull. Basal fractures are

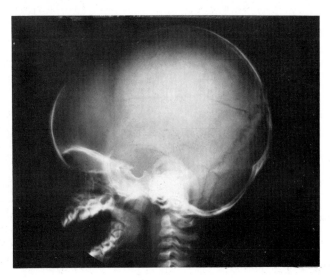

Figure 10.4. Lateral skull radiograph showing a linar fracture across the parietal bone

often difficult to demonstrate radiographically. Linear fractures are slow in healing and may be visible for periods up to 4 years or longer.

(2) *Stellate fractures*—'Star-shaped'. The central point of the fracture is usually due to a local sharp impact. A bone fragment in this central spot may be depressed.

(3) *Depressed fracture*—These are fairly uncommon. A fragment of bone is detached from its surround and depressed or pushed into the brain. This 'fragment' may be comminuted but there can also be a pathway between the fracture and the outside air in which case it is said to be *compound* (*Figure 10.5*). These fractures are often best seen when the fragment is in profile and its degree of depression and position must be assessed. Tangential projections of the skull may therefore be required.

Skull fractures may be directly responsible for injury to the brain. Complications include the following:

(1) Haemorrhage.
(2) Entry of air and infection.
(3) Escape of cerebrospinal fluid.
(4) Cranial nerve damage.

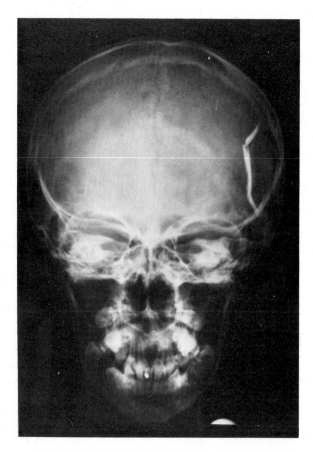

Figure 10.5. A depressed skull fracture in the region of the left parietal bone

(1) *Haemorrhage*—This is the most common complication of a skull fracture, but it should be emphasized that a haematoma can form *without* any bony injury. If a fracture line crosses a vascular groove then this may suggest that an extradural haematoma originating from the damaged vessel could also be present.

(2) *Entry of air and infection*—Pneumocephalus or aerocele means air in the cranial cavity and is most commonly the result of a fracture involving the frontal or ethmoid sinuses. Lateral skull films should always be taken with a horizontal X-ray beam and the patient in the 'brow-up' position so air and air/fluid levels can be best visualized behind the frontal bone. The danger of air entry in any compound fracture of the skull lies in the possibility that it may carry with it bacteria and hence infection. Foreign bodies and fragments of scalp and hair can also admit micro-organisms, with meningitis or cerebral abscess possible outcomes.

(3) *Escape of cerebrospinal fluid*—A compound fracture involving the ethmoid, frontal or sphenoid sinuses may result in *cerebrospinal fluid rhinorrhoea*—escape of fluid down the nose. This is sometimes accompanied by pneumocephalus. A compound fracture of the temporal bone can cause loss of cerebrospinal fluid from the external auditory meatus—*cerebrospinal fluid otorrhoea*.

(4) *Cranial nerve damage*—Cranial nerves may be ruptured by the trauma of a head injury and quite often fractures of the skull base may pass through foramina. Symptoms and effects will depend on which nerve has been damaged. The abducent nerve is occasionally involved in fractures of the skull base; paralysis of this nerve results in a medial squint as the lateral rectus muscle of the eye is affected. If the internal auditory meatus is involved then tearing of the vestibulocochlear nerve will cause deafness.

Tumours and other space-occupying lesions

Until its nature is more accurately determined an *intracranial tumour* may be called a *space-occupying lesion* (a blanket term which can also describe intracranial haematoma or abscess). By definition the lesion 'takes up' space and in the closed box of the skull the increase in volume of contents causes the intracranial pressure to rise. This *raised intracranial pressure* can produce very definite radiological signs, the nature of which usually depends on whether the patient is a child or adult.

In a child widening of the sutures—*suture diastasis*—will occur where the joints have not yet fused. This widening tends to be more obvious at the coronal suture and least prominent at the lambdoid suture. Young infants and neonates with raised intracranial pressure will also have large heads with markedly thin skull vaults. *Hydrocephalus* is the usual cause of raised intracranial pressure in the new-born (*see* page 177).

In adults there may be changes in the radiological appearances. *Erosion* of the lamina dura at the base of the dorsum sellae represents an 'early change' due to raised intracranial pressure. In later stages the whole of the dorsum sellae may disappear. Other signs of an intracranial space-occupying lesion in an adult include the following:

(1) *Mid-line displacement of the pineal gland*—The pineal gland is frequently calcified and because of its situation in the mid-line of the brain its shift can sometimes indicate an intracranial abnormality. The calcified gland can be seen on fronto-occipital projections of the skull. A shift of more than 3 mm to one side of the mid-line is thought to be abnormal.

(2) Presence of an intracranial tumour may be disclosed by its *calcification*. The appearance of the calcification tends to be characteristic for a particular lesion but not all calcification is indicative of pathology (or of a tumour). Structures in the brain that may become normally calcified include the falx cerebri and the pineal gland.

(3) *Abnormal vascular markings* on the bony walls of the skull. An example of this is in a *meningioma* (tumour of the meninges) where the tumour derives part of its blood supply from the middle meningeal artery. The artery (which grooves the lateral wall of the skull) becomes enlarged on the affected side. Its vascular channels consequently become more deepened and thus more obvious on the lateral skull radiograph. The middle meningeal artery passes through the foramen spinosum—so enlargement of this orifice when seen on the SMV projection is another clue to the abnormality.

Tumours of the head (cranium and brain) can be grouped according to their site of origin: (1) intracranial tumours, (2) extracranial tumours, and (3) tumours of the cranial bones.

Intracranial tumours

(a) Primary tumours:

(1) *Gliomas* are relatively common brain tumours arising from nervous tissue.

(2) *Meningiomas*—Tumours arising from the meninges.

(3) *Pituitary adenomas*—As pituitary tumours increase in size they enlarge and erode the pituitary fossa. This is sometimes called 'ballooning' of the sella. Although the appearance is characteristic the radiologist may have to determine whether the changes are due to a tumour or to raised intracranial pressure. Eighty per cent of pituitary tumours are *chromophobe adenomas*—arising from chromophobe cells in the anterior part of the gland. As the tumour enlarges it tends to press on the optic chiasma and affects the patient's sight. (It is now

thought that most of these tumours secrete prolactin and are hence termed *prolactinomas*.) *Acidophil adenoma* of the pituitary gland also causes enlargement of the fossa but it is probably more noteworthy because in adults it will result in *acromegaly*. Radiographs of the skull show thickening and enlargement of the bones of the vault, the sinuses and protrusion of the jaw (*see* Chapter 3).

(4) *Acoustic neuroma* is a common intracranial tumour which acts as a space-occupying lesion causing erosion and expansion of the internal auditory meatus and sometimes erosion of the petrous apex. The patient suffers from nerve deafness on the affected side and, as the seventh cranial nerve is also involved, facial nerve weakness. Often there may be only a minor degree of bone involvement so special radiographic projections are taken to demonstrate this region of the temporal bone.

(5) *Optic glioma* is a rare tumour usually affecting children. It causes enlargement of the optic canal and optic foramen. Changes in the optic foramina and the sphenoid fissure may also indicate the presence of an intraorbital lesion.

(b) Secondary tumours. The brain is a common site for metastatic deposits of tumours, particularly in cases of carcinoma of the bronchus, breast, kidney, colon and nasopharynx.

Extracranial tumours

Erosion of the skull from tumours originating from outside the skull is relatively rare. A *nasopharyngeal carcinoma* can affect the base of the skull and produce bony erosion, usually in the middle fossa. *Glomus jugulare* tumours arise from specialized neuroendocrine tissues located in the region of the jugular bulb. As the tumour grows it tends to erode the bone by pressure. The areas affected are the jugular foramen, inferior aspect of the petrous bone and the middle ear.

Tumours of the bone

These may be primary or secondary. *Primary tumours* of the skull causing bone erosion are uncommon. *Secondary or metastatic tumours* of the skull where bone erosion is produced are very common. Examples are: *secondary carcinoma* from a primary in the lung and *myelomatosis* with its widespread deposits usually involving the vault of the skull.

Hyperostosis

This is thickening of the skull vault and may be generalized or local.

Hyperostosis frontalis interna is a normal condition and is more common in females. There is irregular ridge-like thickening of the inner table of the frontal bone. The irregular mounds of bone project into the cranial cavity. The cause of this is unknown. Generalized hyperostosis also occurs in *Paget's disease* where there is an increase in the thickness of the skull. The bones also become softer and the texture changes so the radiographs show a 'woolly' mottled appearance (*see* Chapter 3). A *meningioma* may also cause hyperostosis in the region of the tumour.

Platybasia and basilar impression

In these conditions the base of the skull appears relatively flattened. Platybasia is said to be present where the *basal angle* is greater than 142 degrees. The basal angle is between the plane of the clivus of the sphenoid (the sloping part behind the dorsum sellae) and the plane of the mid-line of the anterior fossa. Platybasia is most likely to be found in *Paget's disease* and in *osteogenesis imperfecta* (*see* Chapter 3).

Basilar impression or basilar invagination refers to an elevation or 'inward folding' of the floor of the posterior fossa of the skull. It is usually due to some congenital anomaly of the cervical spine such as fusion of the atlas to the occipital condyle or *Klippel–Feil syndrome* (*see* Chapter 8). Other causes include *rheumatoid arthritis* or when a disease process causes softening of the bone as in *Paget's disease* (*Figure 10.6*), *rickets* or *osteomalacia*.

The degree of platybasia and basilar impression can be assessed from plain radiographs of the skull and a number of lines and measurements have been used for this purpose. Tomography in the anteroposterior position will also disclose the relative positions of the atlanto-occipital joints and the skull base.

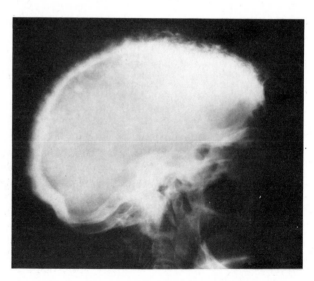

Figure 10.6. A lateral skull radiograph showing the characteristic appearance of Paget's disease. The patient has basilar invagination

Developmental abnormalities

There are several variations in the size and shape of the skull which do not necessarily have any clinical significance. Many descriptive terms are used, for example *dolichocephaly* means that the skull is long in relation to its transverse diameter whereas *brachycephaly* means that it is wide in relation to its length. Note that a skull may be normally asymmetrical—one side is slightly smaller or larger than the other. This can pose problems for an unwary radiographer when the aim is to produce 'non-rotated' frontal or occipital projections of the head!

Craniosynostosis

This is premature closure of one or more cranial sutures. There are several different patterns giving rise to various deformities. This can result in the patient having an 'odd' appearance but in some cases he may also have some neurological disability.

Microcephaly

The skull is very small but the sutures are normal. The condition is due to a failure in the development of the brain.

Craniocleidodysostosis

This is a rare condition where normal ossification of membranous bone is affected. The skull is rather flat and broad and shows prominent suture lines which are sometimes widely separated owing to the lack of bone development. There is also either complete or partial absence of the clavicles (*see* Chapter 6).

Hypertelorism of the orbits

This is an abnormal increase in the interorbital distance which may be associated with craniocleidodysostosis or other bone dysplasias.

Hydrocephalus

Cerebrospinal fluid secreted by the choroid plexuses circulates through the ventricles and cisterns of the brain and around the subarachnoid space of the spinal cord and cerebral hemispheres. It eventually returns to the blood via the arachnoid villi which are situated mainly in the walls of the cerebral venous sinuses. If this flow is obstructed then fluid will accumulate under pressure in the ventricles—*hydrocephalus*. The obstruction may be caused by a tumour but it is more frequently a consequence of some congenital abnormality.

The commonest congenital causes of hydrocephalus are *stenosis* of the aqueduct and *Arnold–Chiari malformation*. In the Arnold–Chiari malformation part of the medulla oblongata and part of the cerebellum lie below the level of the foramen magnum in the spinal canal. The foramen magnum becomes plugged by these structures so that the cerebrospinal fluid is unable to escape through the foramina of Luschka and Magendie and is dammed back. The ventricles and the aqueduct dilate with fluid which continues to be secreted by the choroid plexuses and as intracranial pressure rises the unfused bones of the skull separate. The Arnold–Chiari malformation accompanies *spina bifida* (*see* Chapter 8).

Temporal bones

The temporal bones are included in both the sides and the base of the skull. Important features and elements of the bone are as follows:

(1) The flat *squamous* part forms part of the lateral wall of the cranium.
(2) The *petrous* part of the temporal is wedged between the sphenoid and occipital bones of the skull base. It contains the organs of equilibrium and hearing. The bone forms a covering for the membranous labyrinth (semicircular canals, utricle, saccule and cochlea). The conducting mechanism of hearing (EAM, tympanic membrane, middle ear and its ossicles) also lies in the confines of the petrous temporal. The *internal auditory canal* transmits the vestibulocochlear and facial nerves across the petrous bone in a mediolateral direction and terminating posteriorly just above the jugular foramen. Normally each canal is approximately 10 mm in length.
(3) Extending throughout the posterior part of the temporal bone and into the *mastoid process* is a system of *air cells* which interconnect with each other and the *mastoid antrum*. The antrum is an air sinus which communicates with the middle ear. The air cells can vary greatly in size and extent and are not always comparable on both sides of the skull. In some individuals they are completely absent.
(4) The *styloid process* projects down and forwards from the undersurface of the bone. It gives attachment to certain muscles and ligaments.

Injuries

Fractures of the temporal bone can be restricted to that area or be an extension of a fracture from the skull base or vertex. Radiography can demonstrate the relationship of a fracture line to the facial nerve canal and labyrinth thus helping to assess the possibility of recovery from a resultant facial nerve palsy or deafness.

Barotrauma can also affect the middle ear (*see* Chapter 11).

Other conditions

Infections

Acute mastoiditis—The middle ear communicates with the nasopharynx via the Eustachian tube. Physiologically the tube serves to equalize pressure between the middle ear and the atmosphere but it can also act as a potential route for the spread of infection between the two points. Infection in the middle ear is called *otitis media*. Usually this condition is treated by antibiotics and it spreads no further. If the infection is allowed to develop then the mastoid air cells are also affected.

Chronic mastoiditis—This can occur as a sequel to acute mastoiditis when the infection has failed to resolve. Obliteration of the mastoid air cells now occurs as new bone is formed following the breakdown of the air-cell walls. A *cholesteatoma* is a mass of epithelial cells which has been stimulated to proliferate as a result of the infection of the middle ear or mastoid. This mass erodes the bony walls of the attic, antrum or middle ear and can destroy the ossicular chain. The extent of the erosion can be assessed by *tomography* but some cholesteatomas are not detected by radiography because they cause no bony changes.

Acoustic neuroma

A tumour arising from the sheath of the 8th cranial nerve may expand and produce changes in the internal auditory canal which includes its widening and shortening. Note that there is considerable normal variation in the width and length of the canal and only about 40% are found to be symmetrical in the occipitofrontal projection[2]. (*See* also page 175.)

Congenital abnormalities

Deformities or even absence of part or parts of the hearing/equilibrium apparatus in the petrous bone occur.

Bell's palsy

This is a disorder of the facial nerve with resultant paralysis involving both upper and lower facial muscles and an inability to shut the eye or even to blink on the affected side. The cause of Bell's palsy is unknown and the majority of patients recover spontaneously.

Meniere's syndrome

A group of symptoms—deafness, *vertigo* (dizziness) and *tinnitus* (ringing in the ears)—involving both cochlear and vestibular (8th) nerve endings. The cause is unknown and the severity of the symptoms varies.

Radiographic techniques

Because of the anatomical complexity and spherical structure of the skull a single projection produces a composite picture. Several views are thus needed in order to fulfil diagnostic requirements. Patient positioning tends to be standardized although the selection and number of projections used is subject to departmental variation. Reference must be made to certain anatomical points, lines and planes on the head (*Figure 10.7*). Use of these helps the radiographer to standardize projections.

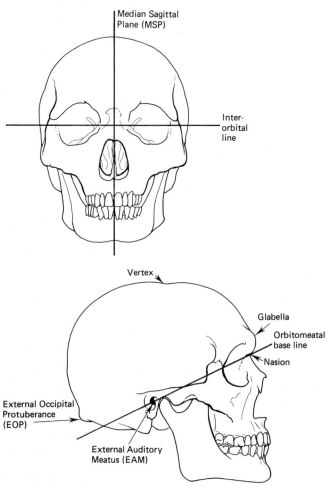

Figure 10.7. Anatomical lines, planes and landmarks that are important in radiography of the head

Median sagittal plane—This divides the skull in the mid-line from front to back.

Interorbital/interpupillary line—This joins the centre of the two orbits. It is at right angles (perpendicular) to the median sagittal plane.

Orbitomeatal base line—The base line or radiographic base line. This joins the outer canthus of the eye to the central point of the EAM. Alternative base lines are available but this is the one used throughout the text.

During radiography, general patient position can be either erect or horizontal depending on preference and patient condition. With very few exceptions a *grid* is always used in radiography of the skull.

The following techniques assume that a conventional horizontal or vertical bucky table is in use. Special techniques have been devised for use with the more specialized or isocentric equipment, e.g. skull table, 'Orbix'. Generally speaking, these are *positioning* methods which will produce similar results to conventional techniques. With the exception of the 'Stockholm C' projection for the temporal bone these special methods are not included.

Some form of *immobilization* device, e.g. bucky band or head clamp, should always be used.

Cranium

Techniques (1–7) include the general survey projections for the cranium. Projections (8–18) include those for localized parts of the cranium.

(1) Occipitofrontal skull

The patient is erect or prone facing the film. The forehead rests on the table. The base line is 90 degrees to the film. The median sagittal plane is perpendicular to the film. Feel the back of the patient's head to check for symmetry. If a skull table is used the patient's face can be seen and centralization of the head can be checked.

Centre—Either (i) in the mid-line so that the central ray emerges through the glabella with the X-ray beam perpendicular to the film. This shows the petrous bones within the orbits on the film. Or (ii) in the mid-line so that the central ray emerges through the nasion. The X-ray beam is angled 20 degrees caudad. The upper border of the petrous bone is seen at the level of the lower border of the orbits on the film.

Alternative techniques—projection (2).

An occipitofrontal projection of the cranium can also be obtained using the methods similar to those outlined in projections (2(ii)) and (2(iii)), page 197.

(2) Fronto-occipital skull

This projection is used where the patient must remain supine or in cases where the back of the skull is of interest. Rest the back of the head on a narrow wedge foam pad. The median sagittal plane is perpendicular to the film. Either of the following may be performed, starting with the base line at 90 degrees to the film:

(i) Raise the chin slightly so the base line is 20 degrees above its original perpendicular position. The orbits will be visible *above* the petrous bones on the film.
(ii) Keep the chin depressed so that the base line remains perpendicular to the film. The petrous bones are seen through the orbits on the film.
Centre: in either case in the mid-line with a 'straight' X-ray tube through the nasion.

In projection (2(ii)), if the patient cannot produce or maintain the position, additional caudal angulation of the tube may be necessary to compensate for the raised base line. Disadvantages of the fronto-occipital alternative include magnification of the frontal bone and orbits. The FFD can be increased to reduce this effect. Note that the radiation dose to the eyes is always higher in a frontal projection of the head.

(3) Lateral skull (head and neck turned)

The patient faces the X-ray table. The head is turned on to the affected side, and the opposite shoulder is raised slightly. The side of the face and head rests against the support. The median sagittal plane is parallel to the film and the interpupillary line is 90 degrees to it. Pads may be needed to support the head and chin in this position.

Centre—Midway between the glabella and the occipital protruberance with a 'straight' X-ray beam. *Both* laterals should be taken.

Some patients, especially elderly with more limited movement of the neck, find maintaining this position difficult. If the interpupillary line is not at 90 degrees to the film a compensatory tube angulation may have to be made to produce a 'true' lateral projection. The direction of the central ray should be parallel to the interpupillary line. If this position proves unsuitable projection (4) should be attempted.

(4) Lateral skull (head and neck remaining straight)

The patient can be supine or erect. If erect, place a 30 × 24 cm cassette and grid in the chest stand cassette holder. The patient is seated in the general lateral position and the median sagittal plane of the head is parallel to the film.

The affected side touches the cassette and grid. If the patient is supine, place a foam pad under the head. The cassette and grid are propped vertically alongside the head.

Centre—As for projection (3), whether the patient is erect or supine. In position (4) the true relationship between the upper cervical spine and skull base is seen.

(5) *Fronto-occipital (F-O) 30 degrees (half axial) skull*

The patient sits or lies with the back of the head touching the table. Place a small foam pad behind the head and depress the chin until the base line is perpendicular to the film. The median sagittal plane is also perpendicular to the film. Angle the X-ray tube 30 degrees caudad.

Centre—In the mid-line through the frontal bone so the central ray emerges through the foramen magnum. The cassette should be displaced downwards to be centralized with the X-ray beam.

Positioning the base line at 90 degrees to the film may be difficult for the patient; additional caudal tube angulation can be used to compensate for a slightly raised base line. Where a skull table is used the table top can be tilted independently of the tube angle. The head and neck can be tilted forwards thus helping to keep the chin depressed.

On the radiograph the front of the skull is projected downwards off the film leaving the structures that form the back of the skull—the foramen magnum, occipital and posterior parietal bones—relatively undistorted. The dorsum sellae is seen within the foramen magnum and the temporal bones lie on either side. If calcified, the pineal gland should lie in the mid-line (provided that there is nothing causing a mid-line shift).

Kyphosis

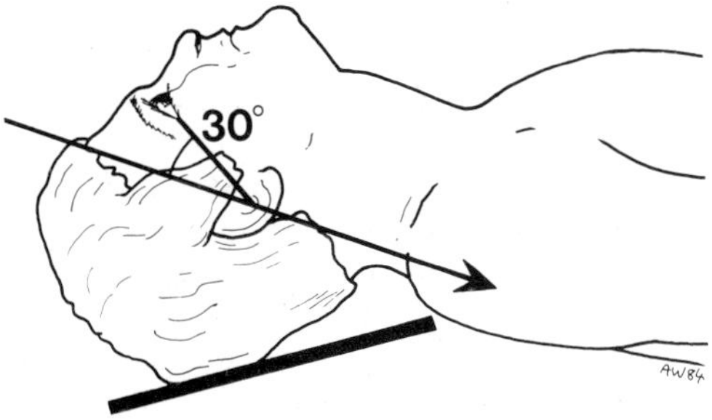

Difficulty is experienced in producing an acceptable F-O 30 degree film in patients with a pronounced spinal curvature (*Figure 10.8*). The patient cannot depress the chin adequately.

To overcome this, lie the patient on the couch. Place a 24 × 30 cm cassette and grid under the head. Support the head and cassette on a pad. The base line is unlikely to be at 90 degrees to the film. Unfortunately, compensatory additional tube angulation projects the occipital bone downwards even further. Since it is usually impossible—owing to the curve of the dorsal spine—to position the cassette low enough, the foramen magnum will not be seen on the film.

Projection (6) may be used as an alternative to the conventional F-O 30 degrees.

(6) *'Reverse' fronto-occipital 30 degrees skull*

The patient sits facing the vertical bucky or skull table with the forehead touching the support. The base line is at 90 degrees to the film. The median sagittal plane is

Figure 10.8. The problem of obtaining a fronto-occipital skull radiograph on a patient who has a 'permanently' extended neck

perpendicular to the film. Angle the tube 30 degrees *cephalad*.

Centre—Below the external occipital protruberance so that the beam emerges through the glabella.

This reverse projection can be done on specialized equipment such as the 'Orbix' so that the patient can remain supine.

The disadvantage of the reverse projection is that the back of the skull is no longer close to the film and will be magnified to some extent.

(7) Submentovertical (SMV/AXIAL) skull

This is easiest for the patient if undertaken using a skull table. The patient lies supine on a couch or trolley, positioned so the shoulders are just beyond the end of the couch. The neck is extended backwards until the vertex of the skull touches the support (*Figure 10.9*).

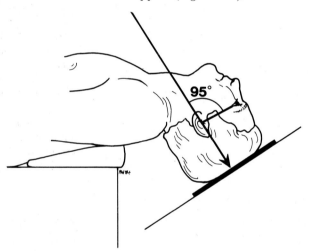

Figure 10.9. Positioning of the patient and angulation of the X-ray beam for the SMV projection (7)

The median sagittal plane is perpendicular to the film. The skull table and head are mutually arranged so that the base line is parallel to the film.

Centre—Between the angles of the jaw in the mid-line with the beam angled 5 degrees cephalad.

Use of a *vertical bucky* is possible but the position is more difficult to achieve and maintain. Sometimes an SMV has to be obtained on a patient who must remain lying on the stretcher or conventional X-ray table and no skull table is available. In this situation pads should be placed under the shoulders and the neck extended as far as possible. A cassette and grid should be placed under the vertex of the skull—if necessary at an angle behind the head—to maintain a parallel relationship with the base line. Centre as above; the base line and central ray should make an angle of 95 degrees.

Unconscious or seriously head-injured patients

The technique of examination must be modified according to the patient's conditions. Several rules are followed:

(1) The patient should be under supervision to detect changes in condition.
(2) The examination should be executed in the shortest possible time.
(3) The patient is examined in the supine position.
(4) Where there is significant patient movement due to cerebral irritation, confusion or disorientation, fast film/screen combinations and short exposure times are required.
(5) The patient's head may need to be held by an assistant. (*Not* by a radiographer.)
(6) Take into consideration *other* injuries the patient may have. Head and neck injuries occur together. A lateral cervical spine radiograph is often routinely requested. Care should be taken if the head has to be lifted. An SMV is not routinely attempted on casualty patients unless sanction has been given.
(7) The laterals should be taken with a horizontal beam (projection (4)). Air/fluid levels may be present inside the cranium. A fluid level in the sphenoid sinuses may be blood which indicates a base fracture.

Some patients with serious head injuries may have to remain in casualty or the intensive care unit for the X-ray examination. In these cases an initial examination may be restricted to two projections—(2(i)) and (4).

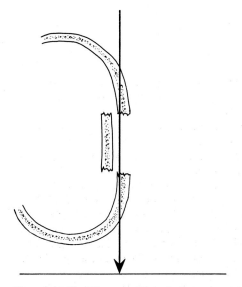

Tangential projections

These are used in the assessment of depressed fractures and also to gain further information about the inner and outer tables of the vault bones. The head is rotated to position the depressed fragment in *profile*. The central ray must be *tangential* to the fragment (*Figure 10.10*).

Alternative imaging in head injuries

Computerized tomography can be used in the investigation of fractures of the skull base, those involving the ethmoid complex and also of the orbit. In cases of depressed fracture, CT allows assessment of possible brain damage. Space-occupying lesions—haematomas—can also be detected by CT and radioisotope scanning.

Ultrasound can detect a shift in mid-line structures but will not in itself determine the *cause* of the shift. (The shift may have been present before the head injury occurred.)

Figure 10.10. The principle of the tangential projection

(8) Pituitary fossa

Additional localized projections are as follows:

(i) *Lateral*—Projection (3) or (4). *Centre:* 2.5 cm above and in front of the uppermost EAM using a collimated beam.

(ii) *Occipitofrontal*—Projection (1). *Centre:* 5 cm below the external occipital protuberance with the X-ray tube angled 10 degrees cephalad using a collimated beam.

(iii) *Fronto-occipital 30 degrees*—Projection (5), using a collimated beam.

Additional information can be obtained using tomography.

(9) Foramen magnum

Additional localized projections are as follows:

(i) *SMV*—Projection (7). *Centre:* Midway between the EAMs using a collimated beam.

(ii) *Fronto-occipital 30 degrees*—Projection (5), using a collimated beam.

(iii) *Lateral*—Projection (3) or (4). *Centre:* 2.5 cm below the EAM uppermost using a collimated beam.

Autotomography (Figure 10.11)

Additional information can be obtained by using this technique. The patient is prone. A cassette and grid are supported vertically at a distance from the head. Request

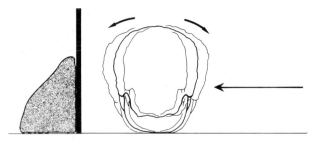

Figure 10.11. The principle of autotomography

the patient to 'say no' by moving his head from side to side 10–15 degrees using the forehead as a pivot. Ask the patient to practise this. Make the exposure using a 3–4 second time. On the radiograph all but the mid-line structures will be blurred, giving the appearance of a mid-line tomogram.

(10) Cribriform plate of the ethmoid

Additional projections are as follows:

(i) *SMV*—Projection (7) if not routinely undertaken.

(ii) *Occipitomental*—Projection (1), Facial bones, page 197. *Centre:* in the mid-line through the vertex just anterior to the EAMs with the X-ray beam angled 40 degrees caudad.

(iii) *Posteroanterior oblique*—From the occipitofrontal position (projection (1)) rotate the head to one side through 45 degrees. Raise the base line through 35 degrees. *Centre:* through the orbit in contact with the film with the beam angled 10 degrees caudad.
Repeat, moving the head in the opposite direction.

In cases of cribriform plate fractures refer to projection (4), Facial bones, page 198.

Crista galli

This is usually shown on the occipitofrontal 20 degrees projection (1(ii)).

(11) Optic foramen (optic canal)

This is the passageway for the optic nerve and ophthalmic artery lying in the lesser wing of the sphenoid bone. A posteroanterior oblique projection is used. The patient is in the occipitofrontal position (projection (1)). The base line is raised through 35 degrees. The head is rotated through 45 degrees, bringing the orbit of the side under examination closest to the film.

Centre—With a horizontal beam directly through the orbit nearest the film.

The foramen is seen in the outer section of the orbit. There are variants of this position but the radiographic principle is the same for each: the central ray must pass directly through the optic foramen.

Repeat the procedure for the other side. The two foramina will be compared, therefore the positioning must be comparable. Additional information can be obtained by using tomography.

(12) Superior orbital fissure

This transmits the oculomotor, trochlear, ophthalmic and abducent nerves. The fissure is demonstrated on the occipitofrontal 20 degrees projection of the skull (1(ii), page 181).

(13) Jugular foramina

These lie at the posterior ends of the petro-occipital suture. Each transmits the internal jugular vein, and the glossopharyngeal, vagus and accessory nerves. Localized projections include:

(i) *Modified SMV*—This shows both foramina; the position is the same as in projection (7).

Centre: midway between the EAMs with the beam angled 20 degrees caudad. Use a narrow rectangular diaphragm.

(ii) *Lateral oblique*—This shows a single foramen. Commence with the head in the true lateral position (projections (3) or (4)). Turn the face slightly towards the film through 15 degrees.
Centre: 2.5 cm above and behind the EAM remote from the film with the beam angled 15 degrees caudad. Repeat the procedure for the other side.

(iii) *Fronto-occipital 30 degrees*—Projection (5), using a narrow rectangular diaphragm. This projection may show bony erosion in the petrous bone.

Additional information can be obtained from tomography and jugular venography.

(14) Foramen rotundum

This transmits the maxillary nerve (a branch of the trigeminal). The foramen can be seen inside the maxillary antrum, below the orbit on the occipitomental projection (projection (1), Facial bones, page 1).

(15) Foramina ovale, lacerum, spinosum

The foramen ovale transmits the mandibular branch of the trigeminal nerve, the foramen lacerum the internal carotid artery and the foramen spinosum the middle meningeal artery. These foramina can be visualized on the SMV projection (7).

Temporal bones

The following list of projections is not claimed to be comprehensive. Several combinations of projection are feasible for the demonstration of the anatomy of the petromastoid portion of the temporal bones.

(16) Middle and inner ear

Additional localized projections are as follows:

(i) Fronto-occipital 35 degrees

As for projection (5) with 5 degrees additional caudal angulation.
Centre—Using a rectangular diaphragm in the mid-line so the beam passes between the EAMs.

(ii) SMV—Projection (7)

Centre—Midway between the EAMs with a rectangular diaphragm.

(iii) Lateral oblique—Projection (13(ii))

Centre—5 cm above and behind the EAM remote from the film with the beam angled 15 degrees caudad.

Repeat for the other side.

(iv) Posteroanterior oblique

This is a version of Stenver's projection. The patient commences in the occipitofrontal position (projection (1)). The head is 'off-centred' 2.5 cm so the orbit of the side of interest is over the cross-lines of the table. The head and neck are tilted axially 15 degrees away from the side of interest. The head is now rotated through 45 degrees, the side of interest remaining closest to the film. The X-ray tube is angled 12 degrees cephalad.

Centre—Midway between the external occipital prot-ruberance and the EAM of the side nearest the X-ray tube.

Repeat for the other side.

(v) 'Stockholm C' projection

A skull table is used. The head is in the true lateral position. The table cross-lines are 2 cm in front of and 1 cm above the EAM. Flex the neck slightly so the base line is at an angle of 5 degrees to the transverse cross-lines.

Centre—With the X-ray tube angled 30 degrees towards the face (from the back of the head) and 10 degrees towards the head (cephalad). Displace the cassette 2 cm upwards in the tray. The grid must be rotated so that the grid slats are parallel to the direction of the angled beam.

The radiograph produced by the 'Stockholm C' projection is similar to that produced with projection (16(iv)).

(vi) Anteroposterior oblique

The head is in the fronto-occipital position (projection (2)) with the base line at 90 degrees to the film. Rotate the head through 45 degrees towards the side of interest. (The petrous temporal of this side is now 90 degrees to the film.)

Centre—5 cm above the outer canthus of the eye remote from the film with the beam angled 45 degrees caudad. The central ray should pass through the EAM nearest the film.

(17) Internal auditory canals

(i) *Transorbital projection*—Position as for projection (2).
Centre: in the mid-line between the orbits using a narrow rectangular beam. The X-ray tube is perpendicular to the film.

This projection can be taken with the head in the occipitofrontal position. Some radiologists consider this to be the most useful projection and measurements of canal dimensions may be taken from the film. Macroradiographic technique can also be undertaken but the radiation dose to the eyes should be considered.

(ii) *Fronto-occipital 35 degrees*—The same comments apply as for projection (16(i)).

(iii) *SMV*—Same comments apply as for projection (16(ii)).

(iv) *Posteroanterior oblique*—Projection (16(iv)) or its variants.

(18) Mastoid complex

The air cells and the mastoid process.

(i) Fronto-occipital 35 degrees

The same comments apply as for projection (16(i)).

(ii) SMV

The same comments apply as for projection (16(ii)).

(iii) Lateral oblique

The head is in the true lateral position (projection (3)). The pinna of the ear next to table top may be folded forwards to avoid superimposition of the soft-tissue shadows on the mastoid area.

Centre—5 cm above and behind the EAM remote from the film with the X-ray tube tilted 25 degrees caudad. This tube angulation can be varied. Repeat for the opposite side.

(iv) Lateral oblique

Position as for projection (13(ii)).

Centre—5 cm above and behind the EAM remote from the film with the X-ray beam angled 15 degrees caudad. The pinna of the ear can be folded forwards as in projection (18(iii)). Repeat for the opposite side.

(v) Profile mastoid process

The tip is superficial and does not require a large exposure. A grid is not necessary. The patient is supine in the fronto-occipital position (projection (2)). The base line is 90 degrees to the film. Rotate the face through 35 degrees away from the side of interest. The aim is to project the mastoid process below the occipital bone and clear of the cervical vertebrae.

Centre—With a 15 degree caudad angle directly over the mastoid process. Repeat for the opposite side.

Tomography

Tomographs are particularly useful in the evaluation of bone changes in the internal auditory canals and in detecting bony destruction in and around the middle ear. The technique is used extensively in the investigation of middle-ear disease, fractures and congenital deformities of the temporal bone.

Computerized tomography

This can detect the extent of bone involvement and destruction in tumours of the region.

References

1. EVANS, K.T. (1977). The radiologists dilemma. *British Journal of Radiology*, **50**, 229–300
2. SUTTON, D. (1980). *A Textbook of Radiology and Imaging*, 3rd edn, p. 988. Edinburgh; Churchill Livingstone

11 The face: facial bones and sinuses

Indications for the X-ray examination

Facial bones

The skeleton of the face can be divided into three parts. The *upper third* above the superior orbital ridges belongs to the cranium. The *middle third* lies between the superior orbital ridges and the occlusal line of the upper teeth. The *lower third* of the face is the mandible.

Bones of the middle third of the face include:

(1) The maxillae and palatine bones above the upper teeth.
(2) The nasal, ethmoid and lacrymal bones between the orbits.
(3) The zygomatic or cheek bones.
(4) The sphenoid and frontal bones of the posterior and upper walls of the orbit.
(5) The paired pterygoid processes of the sphenoid bone lying directly behind the maxillae.

A discussion of dental pathology and radiography is outside the scope of this book.

Facial injuries

Injuries to the middle third of the face are usually inflicted during road-traffic accidents when passengers are thrown forward against a windscreen. As they are often subsidiary to more serious injuries they may be overlooked—particularly as the patient may develop gross oedema of the face, making fractures difficult to diagnose either clinically or radiologically.

The maxillae consist of thin plates or sheets of bone connected together with some parts reinforced to form strong vertical buttresses designed to withstand the stress of mastication. These do not offer much resistance to horizontal forces, and as the thin plates enclose air-filled cavities injury tends to shatter them. The facial bones can fracture in several patterns and in any combination depending on the direction and severity of the blow.

Different methods of classification can be used but it is usual to group the fractures according to the region of the face affected: e.g. fractures of the zygomatic region; fractures of the nasal region; bilateral fractures of the mid-face (Le Fort fractures); and orbital 'blow-out' fractures.

Le Fort fractures

These complex and bilateral mid-face fractures involving several bones produce detached segments of bone that are often freely movable. There are three types:

(1) *Le Fort I*—A horizontal fracture which separates the hard palate and the alveolar process from the middle face (*Figure 11.1*).
(2) *Le Fort II*—The fracture line involves the nasal bones and the orbital floor, passing through walls of the maxillary sinus to the pterygoid plates of the sphenoid (*Figure 11.2*). This separates the mid-portion of the face from the cranium and lateral aspects of the face. If this detached segment is displaced backwards, then in the lateral radiograph the face will have a 'dish-face' appearance.
(3) *Le Fort III*—There is a detachment of the whole of the mid-facial skeleton from the cranial base (*Figure 11.3*). The fracture lines involve the nasal bones at a high level. They cross the medial wall of the orbit, extending into the inferior orbital fissure and continue along the lateral orbital wall to the zygomaticofrontal suture. The zygomatic arch and pterygoid plates are also fractured.

Le Fort fractures can occur in various combinations and sometimes two or all three types can occur simultaneously. Considerable force is required to produce fractures of this magnitude. The patient will have associated soft-tissue

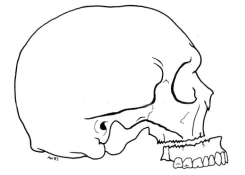

Figure 11.1. Le Fort type I fracture, lateral aspect

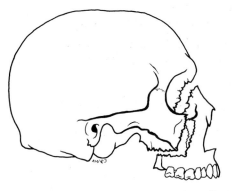

Figure 11.2. Le Fort type II fracture, lateral aspect

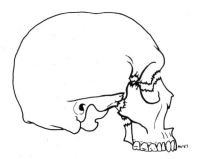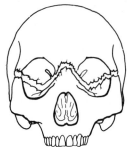

Figure 11.3. Le Fort type III fracture, lateral and frontal aspects

injuries and displacement of the bony segments resulting in haemorrhage or airway obstruction that require urgent surgery.

Orbital 'blow-out' fractures

A direct blow to the eye may cause a fracture of the thin orbital floor without there being any damage to the orbital margins (*Figure 11.4*). The globe of the eye is distorted by the blow and the force is transmitted to the bony walls. As

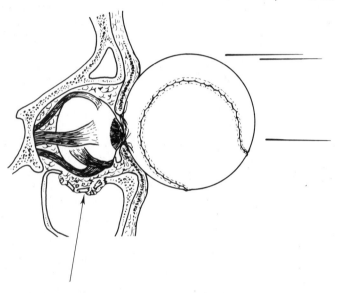

Figure 11.4. The mechanism of the orbital 'blow-out' fracture

the orbital floor is the weakest area it fractures. Periorbital tissue—muscle and fat—is displaced downwards into the maxillary antrum. The lowered position of the eye causes the patient to have double vision—*diplopia*. The most useful radiographic investigation to confirm or assess a blow-out fracture is *tomography*.

Fractures of the mandible

A fracture can occur at any place in the mandible but there are certain sites that are more vulnerable because of their relative inherent weakness. These are:

(1) The condyle neck which is slim.
(2) The mandibular angle which is weakened by the change in direction of the bone grain and often by the presence of an unerupted wisdom tooth.
(3) The body where the tooth sockets weaken the bone—e.g. the canine tooth socket.

Mandible fractures are often compound because they 'open' into the mouth. A *flail mandible* (*Figure 11.5*) is a serious injury where the bone is broken at the symphysis and also

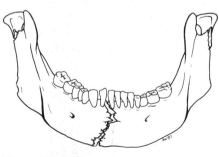

Figure 11.5. Flail mandible

on both sides through the ramus or condyles. These multiple fractures result in loss of bony support for the tongue and the floor of the mouth and thus permit posterior displacement of these structures causing airway obstruction. The patient should either remain sitting or lying on his side and it may be necessary for him to be intubated via the nasopharynx to maintain breathing.

Dislocation of the mandibular condyles

When dislocated the condyle lies in front of the articular eminence of the temporal bone. It can be dislocated on one or both sides. Fracture–dislocation also occurs. The articular disc or meniscus can be damaged following trauma and the joint can subsequently degenerate in a *secondary osteoarthritis* (*see* Chapter 3).

Paranasal sinuses

The sinuses are air-filled bony boxes. Changes in their radiopacity, the thickness or shape of their mucous membrane lining and the state of their bony walls tell the radiologist about their normality.

Infections (sinusitis)

Infection of the sinuses produces swelling of the lining mucous membrane and filling of the cavity with fluid exudate—a product of the inflamed tissues.

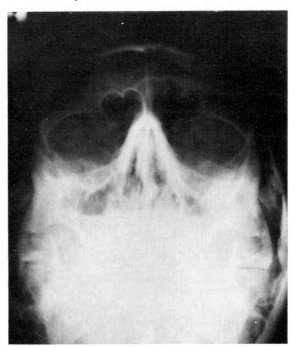

Figure 11.6. An occipitomental radiograph showing fluid levels in the maxillary sinuses

The thickness of the mucosa can be seen on the radiographs but if the sinus is filled with fluid then it will appear uniformly opaque when compared with an unaffected side. Where there is sufficient air and fluid present in the sinus then a *fluid level* will form (*Figure 11.6*). Fluid levels are most easily demonstrated in the maxillary antrum. If infection persists in a sinus when its outlet is blocked then it may become filled with pus—*empyema*. Other conditions can produce changes in the lining mucosa without the formation of fluid levels.

Polypus

This is an outgrowth of mucosa attached to the wall of the nasal cavity or sinus by a stalk. Nasal polyps can occur as a sequel to infective or allergic changes in the mucous membranes.

Barotrauma

This is a form of trauma which may affect the paranasal sinuses (and the mastoid air cells) as a result of alterations in atmospheric pressure. If there is a failure of equalization of pressure in a sinus because of some obstruction of its opening then thickening of its mucosal lining may result. These changes can affect divers or sub-aqua swimmers, for example.

New growths

A tumour of the sinuses is most likely to be a carcinoma—a malignant tumour of the epithelial lining and not of the bone. These most frequently arise in the maxillary antrum or in the ethmoid sinuses. Radiographically the sinus will become opaque and the bony walls will gradually be eroded as the tumour infiltrates and destroys it.

Radiographic techniques

The facial bones (middle third of the face)

The reference lines and planes used in positioning of the head are defined and illustrated in Chapter 10. The comments concerning the use of a grid and immobilizing devices for the skull are equally applicable to techniques for the facial bones. Techniques (1–4) give a general picture of the facial bones. Techniques (5–8) include supplementary projections for localized areas.

(1) Occipitomental facial bones

The patient is erect facing the bucky table. The median sagittal plane is 90 degrees to the film. The chin is raised and rests on the table surface so that the base line makes an angle of 45 degrees with the film.

Centre—With a horizontal X-ray beam so the central ray emerges at the nasion.

On the film the petrous bones are projected below the maxillary sinuses. In using erect positioning with a horizontal X-ray beam, the presence of any fluid levels in the maxillary antra (e.g. presence of blood) may be disclosed. Air may be seen collecting above the orbit in *orbital emphysema* denoting a possible fracture extending into the ethmoid sinuses.

Alternative techniques—projection (2).

(2) Where the patient must remain horizontal

(i) *A 'reverse' occipitomental* can be taken. The patient is supine. The median sagittal plane is perpendicular to the film. The chin is raised (if possible) and the X-ray beam is centred over the upper lip in the mid-line. The X-ray beam should make an angle of 45 degrees with the orbitomeatal base line. A cephalad tube angle may be required. (Backward tilting of the head may not be permissible.) The aim is to project the maxillae above the petrous bones. In the reverse position magnification is inevitable because of the large subject–film distance. It is possible to take this projection using a substantially increased FFD (but *without* a grid); distortion is thereby reduced. The occipitomental projection is always superior to the reverse view. Alternative methods of obtaining these occipitomental projections on an injured patient in the supine position are as follows.

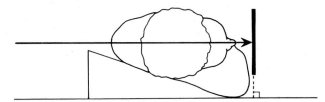

Figure 11.7. Position of the head and the film and the direction of the central ray in projection (2(ii))

(ii) *Occipitomental head turned*—Turn the head and neck over to one side, raising the shoulder so that an occipitomental projection with a horizontal beam can be taken (*Figure 11.7*). The cassette and grid are supported in front of the patient's face with the base line at 45 degrees to the film.

(iii) *Use of special equipment* such as the 'Orbix' where the patient remains supine and the film is positioned in front of the face.

(3) Occipitomental 30 degrees facial bones

The same position is used as in projection (1).

Centre—With the X-ray tube angled 30 degrees caudally, through the vertex so the central ray emerges in the mid-line at the level of the lower orbital margins.

The cassette must be displaced well down. The exposure should be increased from projection (1). The occipitomental 30 degrees projection gives further information about the lower orbital margins and zygoma. With the base line at 45 degrees this projection may be thought to be 'over-tilted'. It may be preferable to rest both chin and tip of nose on the table thus reducing the base line angle. Note that various degrees of tube tilt can be used with a conventional occipitomental position. Some facial surgeons recommend that *no* 'reverse' of the occipitomental 30 degrees position be attempted as the degree of distortion becomes too great to be acceptable.

(4) Lateral facial bones

The patient is erect, facing the vertical bucky table. The head and body are rotated until the affected side of the face is nearest the film and rests on the table. The median sagittal plane is parallel to the film. The interpupillary line is perpendicular to the film.

Centre—With a horizontal beam over the zygomatic bone.

The exposure needed is approximately 10 kVp less than for a lateral skull. A horizontal beam should always be used for the lateral. This may show fluid levels in a sinus, air fluid levels inside the cranium (indicating a cribriform plate fracture). If the patient must remain supine then the cassette and grid are propped by the side of the face. Other positioning criteria remain the same.

Injured patients

Where serious injuries of the face have been sustained, speed and accuracy of technique are vital. The patient may have to be intubated by an anaesthetist as normal breathing may become impossible. Films should be obtained before inhalation takes place wherever possible.

Panoramic zonography

Specialized equipment such as the Siemens 'Zonarc' can produce panoramic radiographs (tomograms) of the facial bones. Films produced can supplement or replace conventional radiography.

(5) Zygomatic arches

Either of the following may be used.

(i) *Fronto-occipital 30 degrees 'jug handle' view*—Position as for projection (5), page 183. Collimate the beam to a rectangle. *Centre:* above the nasion so that the beam passes on either side through the arches. The exposure must be reduced by 15 kVp from a conventional fronto-occipital 30 degrees (projection (5), page 183).

(ii) *Submentovertical*—Position as for projection (7), page 184.

Centre—In the mid-line between the mandibular bodies. Collimate the beam to include the arches, reducing the exposure appropriately.

(6) Nasal bones

(i) *Occipitomental*—As for projection (1). Collimate the beam to the nasal area. Any deviation in the bony septum is seen.

(ii) *Lateral*—The side of the face rests against a cassette or non-screen film. The median sagittal plane is parallel to the film. The interpupillary line is 90 degrees to the film. *Centre:* with a horizontal beam over the root of the nose. The FFD can be increased to compensate for the larger subject–film distance. The lateral is the most useful projection.

(iii) *Superoinferior (Figure 11.8)*—The patient is seated upright. An occlusal film is placed in the mouth, tube side uppermost. Two-thirds of the film lies outside the mouth. The occlusal plane (biting plane) is parallel to the floor. The X-ray beam is directed from above the head in an almost vertical direction to pass through the root of the nose. The patient should wear a lead rubber apron. If the patient has a prominent brow or teeth this projection is not possible.

(iv) *Tomography* can be used for the nasoethmoid complex to determine the extent of a fracture.

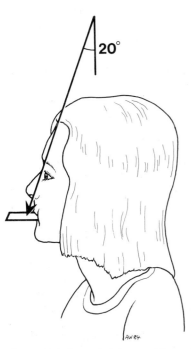

Figure 11.8. Superoinferior nasal bones (projection (6(iii))

(7) Orbits

The orbits are shown on the following projections:

(i) Occipitomental (1).
(ii) Occipitomental 30 degrees (3).
(iii) Lateral (4).
(iv) Occipitofrontal 20 degrees (projection (1(ii)), page 181).

The beam can be collimated to include just the orbits. The following may also be used:

(v) Posteroanterior obliques, for the optic foramina (projection (11), page 187).
(vi) Tomography.

(8) Maxillae

These projections give information concerning minor injuries.

(i) Obliques

The patient faces the vertical bucky. The orbitomeatal base line is raised 10 degrees from the horizontal. The head is rotated through 40 degrees to either side in turn. The nose, forehead and chin are in contact with the table.

Centre—Below the mastoid process remote from the film with the X-ray beam angled 10 degrees cephalad.

(ii) Occlusal films

These demonstrate the alveolar part of the maxilla and hard palate.

(a) Central occlusal—An occlusal cassette is placed in the mouth, short axis cross-wise. The occlusal plane (biting plane) is parallel to the floor. *Centre:* through the vertex with the X-ray tube angled 10 degrees forwards from the vertical to the centre of the cassette.

(b) Angled occlusal—Same position of patient. A non-screen occlusal pack is placed short axis cross-wise in the mouth and pushed back as far as possible. *Centre:* through the tip of the nose with the tube angled 15 degrees backwards from the vertical to the centre of the cassette.

(c) Oblique occlusal—The film is placed long axis cross-wise in the mouth. The beam is directed 25 degrees from the vertical: from the lateral aspect of the face towards the median plane. *Centre:* to just below the outer canthus of the eye, to right and left sides in turn.

Paranasal sinuses

Projections of the paranasal sinuses must be standardized as far as possible so that they are reproducible and thus easily compared. A sinus protractor or similar angle-measuring device can be used when the head is positioned. Collimation of the beam is of special importance and a beam limiting device—usually a cone—is used.

A secondary radiation grid is usually used in sinus radiography but some radiologists can tolerate the 'grey' image of a non-grid technique. The number of projections taken during a routine examination can vary. The minimum is two. Positioning is usually *erect*.

(9) Occipitomental sinuses

The same position in projection (1) is used, with the patient erect.

Centre—In the mid-line so the central ray emerges at the lower border of the orbits using a horizontal X-ray beam.

The petrous bones must be projected below the lower border of the maxillary antra. If they are not then the head is 'undertilted'. If movement of the neck is restricted a compensatory caudal angulation will be needed. If the chin is raised too far then the teeth may obscure the lower antra. The latter tends to occur more readily in children.

The occipitomental projection shows the *maxillary antra*. If the mouth is kept open the *sphenoid sinuses* and *nasopharynx* are seen (especially in an edentulous patient). The *frontal* sinuses are shown but are foreshortened.

Fluid levels

With a horizontal beam, fluid levels in the antra may be shown. For further proof that an opacity is fluid and not mucosal thickening, repeat the occipitomental film but tilt the head and neck to one side through 30 degrees. The fluid will 'settle' because of gravity in a direction parallel to the floor.

(10) Occipitofrontal sinuses

Position as for the occipitofrontal skull (projection (1), page 181).

Centre—Either (i) with the X-ray tube angled caudally between 10 and 15 degrees above the external occipital protruberance to emerge through the nasion. This demonstrates the *frontal sinuses* and the *anterior ethmoids* which are projected above the sphenoid sinuses. *Or* (ii) with a horizontal X-ray beam 4 cm below the external occipital protruberance towards the maxillary sinuses. This demonstrates the *maxillary sinuses* below the level of the petrous temporals. The sphenoid sinuses are superimposed on the anterior ethmoids. *Or* (iii) with a 10 degree cephalad angle towards the nasion. This projects the *sphenoid* sinuses above the ethmoids to be superimposed on the frontal bone.

Fluid levels frontal sinuses

These can be confirmed by the following projection. With the patient supine, the head is turned through 90 degrees (one shoulder is raised). A cassette is propped vertically in front of the face. The median sagittal plane is 90 degrees to the film and parallel to the table top.

Centre as for the occipitofrontal 15 degree projection (10(i)) except using a horizontal beam.

(11) Lateral sinuses

Position as for the lateral skull (projection (3), page 182).

Centre—2.5 cm from the outer canthus of the eye along the base line using a horizontal X-ray beam.

All groups of sinuses are shown but the pairs are superimposed.

(12) Submentovertical sinuses

Position as for the submentovertical skull (projection (7), page 184).

Centre—As for projection (7), page 184.

This demonstrates the *sphenoid* sinuses, the *posterior ethmoids* and also the maxillary antra and orbital walls.

Plan projection, frontal sinuses

The patient position remains the same as in projection (12). Centre inside the arch of the mandible so the central ray passes tangentially through the frontal sinuses.

(13) Posteroanterior oblique sinuses

The patient sits facing the bucky table. The chin is raised so that the base line is 30 degrees from the horizontal. The head is rotated to right and left sides in turn so that the median sagittal plane makes an angle of 40 degrees with the film. The patient's nose, chin and cheek bone touch the table surface.

Centre—With a horizontal beam directly through the orbit nearest the film.

The *posterior ethmoids* are projected through the orbit. The *optic foramen* may also be shown.

Tomography

Conventional tomography has importance in detecting fractures, foreign bodies and bone destruction of the sinus walls in neoplastic disease. *Computerized tomography* can also show the extent of soft-tissue masses and orbital invasion.

Mandible

Fractures can occur on the side of the mandible opposite to that which received the blow—*contre coup* injury—and the mandible can also often fracture in more than one place, therefore it is important that both sides should be adequately demonstrated. Lateral and lateral oblique projections of both sides should be taken for comparison (projections (17, 18 and 19)). If the patient has no teeth, i.e. is edentulous, then the exposure may need to be reduced from the normal situation. Lateral and lateral oblique projections of the mandible can be taken without a secondary radiation grid.

(14) Posteroanterior mandible

Position as for an occipitofrontal skull projection (page 181).

Centre—In the mid-line 7.5 cm below the external occipital protruberance.

This projection shows the whole mandible and demonstrates displacement of fragments in fractures.

Alternative technique—projection (15).

(15) Anteroposterior mandible

Place the head on a small pad to bring the base line 90 degrees to the film. It may not be possible for the patient to depress the chin so if the base line remains slightly raised then this is acceptable.

Centre—In the mid-line over the lower lip.

(16) Lateral mandible

With the patient seated in a chair, ask him to support a cassette by the side of the face. The cassette should be parallel to the median sagittal plane and 90 degrees to the interorbital line. Raise the chin slightly to bring the rami away from the cervical spine.

Centre—4 cm behind the symphysis menti with a horizontal X-ray beam.

Both sides of the mandibular arch are superimposed, but any displaced fracture fragments may be demonstrated. Further projections are needed to separate the two sides of the bone.

(17) Lateral oblique mandible

Arrange the patient and cassette as for projection (16). Now turn the face towards the cassette to bring the body of the mandible parallel to the film, keeping the chin raised (*Figure*

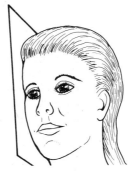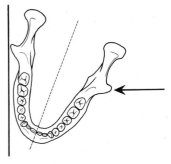

Figure 11.9. The first stage of the positioning in projection (17)—turning the face towards the cassette so that the body of the mandible is parallel to the film

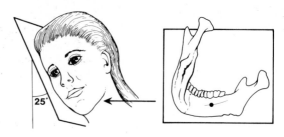

Figure 11.10. Positioning of patient and cassette and direction of the central ray in projection (17(i))

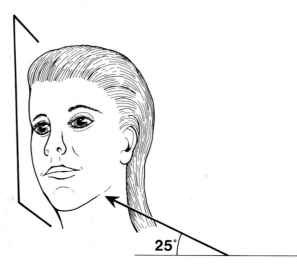

Figure 11.11. Position of patient and cassette in projection (17(ii))

11.9). The X-ray beam is perpendicular to the film. To separate the two sides of the jaw: either (i) tilt both head and cassette over to one side by 25 degrees, using a horizontal X-ray tube (*Figure 11.10*) (*centre:* 5 cm below the angle of the jaw on the side nearest the X-ray tube); or (ii) keep the head straight (*Figure 11.11*) (*centre:* 5 cm below the angle of the jaw but angle the X-ray tube 25 degrees cephalad).

Alternative techniques—projections (18 and 19).

(18) Where the patient remains supine and cannot turn the head

Prop the cassette vertically alongside the face. The head should rest on a foam pad to raise it from the table. Raise the chin if possible. Keep the median sagittal plane parallel to the film and the interorbital line 90 degrees to the film.

Centre—5 cm below the angle of the jaw remote from the film with the X-ray beam angled cephalad 25–30 degrees.

The shoulder nearest the X-ray tube may obstruct the X-ray beam.

(19) If the patient can turn the head and neck

From the supine position the head and neck are rotated towards the side of interest. Raise the opposite shoulder on a pillow. A cassette is supported beneath the face, the median sagittal plane being parallel to the film.

Centre—5 cm below the angle of the jaw remote from the film. The tube is angled 30 degrees cephalad from the vertical and should make an angle of 60 degrees with the cassette.

(20) Submentovertical

Position and centre as for the submentovertical skull (projection (7), page 184).

Collar radiography

A reverse projection to (20) except using special cassette with a cut-out section to place beneath the chin. The beam is directed from above the vertex towards the mandible. This produces a 'plan projection' of the bone—as does projection (20).

(21) Occlusal projections

These are undertaken for a more localized picture of the central mandible. These may show small fractures and any involvement with the teeth. The non-screen occlusal pack is placed and held between the teeth, long axis cross-wise. The X-ray tube side is downwards.

Centre—To the submental aspect of the jaw. The beam should be at right angles to the film.

A dental X-ray set is more convenient but conventional equipment can be used. (It may not always be possible to introduce a film into the mouth if there are injuries to the soft tissues.)

Symphysis menti localized

The same film and patient position is adjusted to 45 degrees.

Centre—To the point of the chin. The angle between the occlusal plane (film) and tube is adjusted to 45 degrees.

(22) Symphysis menti

From the occipitofrontal position (projection (1), page 181) rotate the head through 20 degrees to either side in turn.

Centre—5 cm lateral to the cervical spinous processes and directly through the symphysis menti for the right and left sides in turn. Reduce the exposure from the posteroanterior mandible projection (14). *See* also occlusal projections (21).

(23) Angle of mandible

In the oblique position (22) the angle of mandible nearest the film may be disclosed.

Orthopantomography

Produces a panoramic projection of the mandible and teeth. The film produced is a *tomogram* and a fracture may be missed if the only examination performed uses this technique. The orthopantomogram is very useful, however, and complements 'plain' radiographs.

Temporomandibular joints (TMJs)

When the mouth is opened the condyle of the mandible glides forwards on to the condylar eminence of the temporal bone. By moving the joint in this fashion the radiographer can locate it when touching the patient's face.

(24) Lateral oblique TMJ

In a true lateral projection both joints would be superimposed and obscured by the temporal bones. This projection separates the two sides while the subject remains close to the film. Position as for the lateral skull (projection (3), page 182). Immobilize the head. Three separate exposures for each side are made with the mouth (i) open; (ii) closed; and (iii) teeth clenched together. Explain the procedure carefully to the patient. Use a non-opaque bite block for (i).

Centre—5 cm above the joint remote from the film. The X-ray beam is angled 25 degrees caudad. (In some patients 30 degrees is required.) Collimate the beam. Repeat the procedure for the other side.

These projections may be taken without a grid. The films should be carefully marked.

Alternative technique—projection (25).

Projection (25)

The patient is erect, facing the bucky table. Turn the head so the side of interest touches the table surface. The median sagittal plane is parallel to the film. The interorbital line is 90 degrees to the film. Now the face is rotated through 20 degrees towards the bucky table.

Centre—Towards the TMJ in contact with the table with the beam angled 20 degrees cephalad.

The exposure can be made with the mouth open and closed. Repeat for the other side.

(26) Transpharyngeal projection

This shows the condylar head free from overlying bone structures. The projection is taken through the sigmoid notch (between coronoid process and condyle) of the opposite side of the mandible, across the nasopharyngeal air space. The head is in the true lateral position with a cassette held by the patient against the side of the face. The X-ray tube (dental) is perpendicular to the median sagittal plane. The beam is then angled 5 degrees cephalad and 5 degrees in a posterior direction.

Centre—With the mouth open, to the sigmoid notch of the uppermost side 2.5 cm below the zygomatic arch; and 5 cm anterior to the tragus.

Repeat for the other side.

(27) 'Short distance' technique

With a very short FFD the diverging beam magnifies objects near its source to a far greater extent than an object placed very close to the film. Using dental equipment the patient and cassette are positioned as in projection (26). Keep the mouth closed. The dental X-ray tube cone is positioned touching the uppermost TMJ. The beam is perpendicular to the film and the median sagittal plane.

(28) 'Through orbit' projection

The patient is supine or erect facing the X-ray tube. The orbitomeatal base line is 90 degrees to the film. The median sagittal plane is perpendicular to the film. Rotate the face through 5 degrees towards the affected side. Keep the mouth closed.

Centre—With the X-ray tube angled 10 degrees caudad through the centre of the orbit of the side of interest (nearest the film).

Repeat for the opposite side.

(29) Fronto-occipital both joints

The patient's head is in the fronto-occipital position (projection (2), page 182). A non-opaque bite block should be used to keep the mouth open.

Centre—Above the glabella, in the mid-line with the beam angled 30–35 degrees caudad.

This projection can be taken with the mouth closed.

(30) Occipitofrontal both joints

The patient's head is in the occipitofrontal position (projection (1), page 181). The mouth can be open or closed or the lower jaw protruded.

Centre—7.5 cm below the base line to a point midway between the TMJs with the beam angled 10 degrees cephalad.

Tomography

This is undertaken where 'plain' radiographs have failed to demonstrate the joints. Tomography is usually undertaken with the patient's head in the lateral position. Orthopanto-mography is also useful, especially in cases of injury where a film may be required fairly rapidly.

12   The skeletal survey

The skeletal survey is an examination where radiographs are taken of several areas of the body. The aim of these is to give a complete radiological picture of any given condition involving bony changes and also to monitor progress of changes over a period of time.

Areas of the body included in any survey, selection of projections and frequency of repetition of the examination will always vary according to department and radiologist. Specification of radiographic projections is further hindered because a given pathological condition will affect different individuals in different ways. However, often only one projection is taken of each respective area: e.g. skull and spine, a lateral; long bones, an anteroposterior; hands, a posteroanterior.

When surveys are to be repeated to assess change in radiographic appearances and thus change in the pathological condition, comparability in the standard of work is essential. For example, alterations in bone mineralization density may be masked by changes in exposure factors. Records should be kept if progress is to be followed accurately.

Examples of radiographic skeletal surveys

Further information about the following pathological conditions can be obtained from Chapter 3.

Osteomalacia—Pelvis, thorax, long bones.

Rickets—Long bones, including the wrist and ankle joints. In 'advanced cases', thorax and skull.

Acromegaly—Hands, skull and face, chest, vertebral column, lateral projection of the heels (the thickness of the heel pad may increase).

Hyperparathyroidism—Hands, skull (for mottled areas of deossification), orthopantomogram (loss of lamina dura), lateral calcaneus (resorption of bone in an area subject to stress). 'Advanced cases' may additionally require radiographs of long bones, pelvis, lumbar and dorsal vertebrae.

Hypothyroidism in children—Pelvis, knees, hands, skull.

Osteoporosis—Lumbar and thoracic vertebrae, pelvis, hands and feet.

Paget's disease of bone—Skull, long bones, pelvis, vertebral column.

Osteopetrosis—pelvis, long bones, thorax.

Osteogenesis imperfecta—Infants, radiographs of whole body; older child, long bones, pelvis.

Renal dialysis patients—Full skeletal survey once yearly: pelvis, long bones, thorax, hands, feet, dorsal and lumbar vertebrae, skull. A more limited skeletal survey may be undertaken at 6-monthly intervals between the yearly survey: pelvis, thorax, hands and feet.

Secondary neoplastic disease—Whole spine, skull, pelvis, long bones, thorax. Radioisotope scintigraphy (*see* Chapters 1 and 4) may be used as an alternative to radiography.

Divers and compressed air workers[1]

Individuals exposed to or decompressed from a high ambient pressure may suffer from a disease known as dysbaric necrosis. This occurs as a result of infarcts of bone or bone marrow. Bone cells are deprived of blood supply—they die and result in lesions in the head, neck or shaft of the major long bones. If the lesions involve the articular surface of a major joint osteoarthritis may result.

Affected areas become visible radiographically when new bone is laid down on dead trabeculae and physical density increases. These dense areas may be vague and ill defined therefore high-detail radiographs are vital.

Lesions can occur unilaterally or bilaterally; there is no set pattern.

Areas affected—Head, neck, proximal shaft of humerus and femur; distal end of femur; proximal tibia; elbow and ankle areas (not routinely included in the skeletal survey).

Frequency of survey—Every 6-months during high-pressure work. Annually for 2 years after ceasing to work.

Films—Anteroposterior heads and upper shafts both humeri, femora (not pelvis); anteroposterior and lateral distal two-thirds of both femora and proximal one-third tibia and fibula.

Shoulder radiographs—These must show articular surface of humeral head unobscured by overlying bony structures. Patient supine, rotate 45 degrees to side of examination. Blade of scapula parallel to table. Support raised side. Arm under examination is straight, supinated and abducted 10 degrees. An extending pull to the arm is applied so humeral head is clear of acromion. *Centre:* beam vertical. Over head of humerus. Expose on arrested respiration using a bucky grid. All films must be adequately penetrated (using 5–10 kV above normal).

Battered baby syndrome

A euphemism for this phrase is 'non-accidental' injury to children. Radiographic evidence is fairly specific and used with clinical history to establish a diagnosis. The child may have several injuries in various stages of healing—a skeletal survey is required which may involve radiographing areas of the body that the parents and child are not complaining about. Tact and diplomacy are required in dealing with these patients, who will be accompanied by parents.

Skull fractures are fairly common. The child may have fractures of limb bones but as the periosteum in young children is fairly loosely attached and can be separated from the bone by a direct force, e.g. twisting of the limb, radiographs of long bones in children who have suffered battering may show elevation of the periosteum. Immediately after injury this periosteum remains radiolucent; 2–3 weeks after injury calcium is deposited on the under-surface of the periosteum, making it visible on the films. If further injury occurs during this time or if the initial injury tears the periosteum, callus may form outside the periosteum. After re-union the bone is remodelled to its original form but the cortex may be thickened.

Films—Skull (anteroposterior or posteroanterior, half axial, lateral). Anteroposterior of all long bones, including wrist and ankle joint. Anteroposterior thorax, abdomen, pelvis.

Toddling fractures

These can occur in the long bones of young toddlers, particularly in the tibiae, but these are mostly self-inflicted injuries due to unsteadiness causing the child to bump or fall on to objects. These fractures are always localized and can be excluded radiographically from a 'battered baby syndrome' classification.

Reference

1. MEDICAL RESEARCH COUNCIL DECOMPRESSION SICKNESS PANEL (1981). Divers and compressed air workers. *Radiography*, June, **47**, 141.

Further reading

Anatomy

BERESFORD, W.A. (1977). *Lecture Notes on Histology*, 2nd edn. Oxford; Blackwell.

BRYAN, G.J. (1982). *Johnson and Kennedy Radiographic Skeletal Anatomy*, 2nd edn. Edinburgh; Churchill Livingstone.

GRAYS ANATOMY (1980). 36th edn. Ed. by Williams, P.L. and Warwick, R. Edinburgh; Longman.

SIMON, G. and HAMILTON, W.J. (1978). *X-ray Anatomy*. London; Butterworths.

Orthopaedics

ASTON, J.R. (1976). *A Short Textbook of Orthopaedics and Traumatology*, 2nd edn. London; Hodder and Stoughton.

DUCKWORTH, T. (1980). *Lecture Notes on Orthopaedics and Fractures*. Oxford; Blackwell.

MONK, C.J.E. (1981). *Orthopaedics for Undergraduates*. Oxford University Press.

Pathology

ANDERSON, J.R. (Ed.) (1980). *Muir's Textbook of Pathology*, 11th edn. London; Arnold.

CRAWFORD ADAMS, J. (1972). *Outline of Fractures*, 6th edn. Edinburgh; Churchill Livingstone.

DEL REGATO, J.A. and SPJUT, H.J. (1977). *Cancer*, 5th edn. St Louis; Mosby.

Radiography

CLARK, K.C. (1977). *Positioning in Radiography*, 9th edn. London; Heinemann.

GYLL, C. (1977). *A Handbook of Paediatric Radiography*. Oxford; Blackwell.

KIMBER, P.M. (1983). *Radiography of the Head*. Edinburgh; Churchill Livingstone.

STRIPP, W.J. (1979). *Special Techniques in Orthopaedic Radiography*. Edinburgh; Churchill Livingstone.

Radiology

EDEIKEN, J. and HODES, P.J. (1973). *Roentgen Diagnosis of Diseases of Bone*. Baltimore; Williams and Wilkins.

FORRESTER, D.M. and NESSON, J.W. (1973). *The Radiology of Joint Disease*. Philadelphia; Saunders.

GRECH, P. (1981). *Casualty Radiology*. London; Chapman and Hall.

GREENFIELD, G.B. (1975). *Radiology of Bone Diseases*, 2nd edn. Philadelphia; Lippincott.

ROGERS, L.F. (1982). *Radiology of Skeletal Trauma*. New York; Churchill Livingstone.

SUTTON, D. (1980). *A Textbook of Radiology and Imaging*, 3rd edn. Edinburgh; Churchill Livingstone.

TRAPNELL, D.H. (1967). *Principles of X-ray Diagnosis*. London; Butterworths.

Index